CANCER ETIOLOGY, DIAGNOSIS AND TREATMENTS

CANCER STEM CELLS IN LUNG CANCER

CANCER ETIOLOGY, DIAGNOSIS AND TREATMENTS

Additional books in this series can be found on Nova's website under the Series tab.

Additional E-books in this series can be found on Nova's website under the E-books tab.

CANCER ETIOLOGY, DIAGNOSIS AND TREATMENTS

CANCER STEM CELLS IN LUNG CANCER

KOJI OKUDELA,
AKIRA KATAYAMA,
NORIYUKI NAGAHARA,
AND
HITOSHI KITAMURA

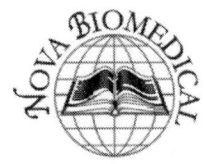

Nova Biomedical Books
New York

Copyright © 2011 by Nova Science Publishers, Inc.

All rights reserved. No part of this book may be reproduced, stored in a retrieval system or transmitted in any form or by any means: electronic, electrostatic, magnetic, tape, mechanical photocopying, recording or otherwise without the written permission of the Publisher.

For permission to use material from this book please contact us:
Telephone 631-231-7269; Fax 631-231-8175
Web Site: http://www.novapublishers.com

NOTICE TO THE READER
The Publisher has taken reasonable care in the preparation of this book, but makes no expressed or implied warranty of any kind and assumes no responsibility for any errors or omissions. No liability is assumed for incidental or consequential damages in connection with or arising out of information contained in this book. The Publisher shall not be liable for any special, consequential, or exemplary damages resulting, in whole or in part, from the readers' use of, or reliance upon, this material.

Independent verification should be sought for any data, advice or recommendations contained in this book. In addition, no responsibility is assumed by the publisher for any injury and/or damage to persons or property arising from any methods, products, instructions, ideas or otherwise contained in this publication.

This publication is designed to provide accurate and authoritative information with regard to the subject matter covered herein. It is sold with the clear understanding that the Publisher is not engaged in rendering legal or any other professional services. If legal or any other expert assistance is required, the services of a competent person should be sought. FROM A DECLARATION OF PARTICIPANTS JOINTLY ADOPTED BY A COMMITTEE OF THE AMERICAN BAR ASSOCIATION AND A COMMITTEE OF PUBLISHERS.

Library of Congress Cataloging-in-Publication Data
Cancer stem cells in lung cancer / Koji Okudela ... [et al.].
   p. ; cm.
  Includes bibliographical references and index.
  ISBN 978-1-61728-295-9 (softcover)
  1. Lungs--Cancer--Pathophysiology. 2. Cancer cells. 3. Stem cells. I. Okudela, Koji.
  [DNLM: 1. Lung Neoplasms--physiopathology. 2. Neoplastic Stem Cells--physiology. 3. Aldehyde Dehydrogenase--physiology. 4. Antigens, CD--physiology. WF 658 C2159 2010]
  RC280.L8C367 2010
  616.99'424--dc22
                        2010022685

Published by Nova Science Publishers, Inc. ✦ *New York*

Contents

Preface		vii
Abbreviations		ix
Chapter I	Introduction	1
Chapter II	Stem Cells in Healthy and Injured Lung	5
Chapter III	Origin of CSCs in Lung Cancers	7
Chapter IV	CD133	13
Chapter V	Side Population	15
Chapter VI	Aldehyde Dehydrogenase	17
Chapter VII	Other Lung CSC Markers	19
Chapter VIII	Signaling Pathways in CSCs of Lung Cancers	21
Chapter IX	Other Signaling Pathways and Transcription Factors in Lung CSCs	23
Chapter X	CSC Niche	25
Chapter XI	Brief Summary of Lung CSC Markers and Potential Problems	27
Chapter XII	ALDH mRNA Expression - Its Correlation with the Most Common CSC Marker CD133	31
Chapter XIII	ALDH Activity in Lung Cancer Cell Lines	35
Chapter XIV	Primary Structure of ALDH1A1 mRNA	39
Chapter XV	Post-translational Modification of ALDH1A1 Protein	41

Chapter XVI	ALDH Protein Expression in Primary Lung Cancers	43
Chapter XVII	Conclusion	47
Acknowledgments		49
References		51
Index		61

Preface

The cancer stem cell (CSC) theory is currently central to the field of cancer research, because it is not only a matter of academic interest but also crucial in cancer therapy. CSCs share a variety of biological properties with normal somatic stem cells in terms of self-renewal, the propagation of differentiated progeny, the expression of specific cell markers and stem cell genes, and the utilization of common signaling pathways and the stem cell niche. However, CSCs differ from normal stem cells in their tumorigenic activity. In this book, we review hitherto described study results and refer to some excellent review articles to understand the basic properties of CSCs. In addition, we focus upon CSCs of lung cancers, since lung cancer is still increasing in incidence worldwide and remains the leading cause of cancer deaths. Understanding the properties of, and exploring cell markers and signaling pathways specific to CSCs of lung cancers will lead to progress in therapy, intervention, and improvement of the prognosisof patients with lung cancer. In the near future, the evaluation of CSCs may be a routine part of practical diagnostic pathology.

Keywords: Cancer stem cell; Small cell lung carcinoma; Non-small cell lung carcinoma.

Abbreviations

SCLC: small cell lung carcinoma;
NSCLC: non-small cell lung carcinoma;
SQC: squamous cell carcinoma;
ADC: adenocarcinoma;
LCC: large cell carcinoma;
RB: retinoblastoma;
TP53: tumor protein 53;
EGFR: epidermal growth factor receptor;
ASCL1: achaete-scute complex homolog 1;
TTF-1: thyroid transcription factor-1;
ALDH: aldehyde dehydrogenase;
CSC: cancer stem cell;
ABCG2: ATP binding cassette transporter superfamily member G2;
CIC: cancer initiating cell;
SP: side population;
FACS: fluorescence activating cell sorting;
UV: ultraviolet;
uPAR: urokinase plasminogen activator receptor;
uPA: urokinase plasminogen activator;
Shh: Sonic hedgehog;
BMP: bone morphogenetic protein;
Bmi1: B cell-specific Mo-MuLV integration site 1;
PODXL-1: podocalyxin-like protein 1;
RT-PCR: reverse transcription polymerase chain reaction;
mRNA, messenger ribonucleic acid;
cDNA; complementary deoxyribonucleic acid;
siRNA: small interfering RNA;
PI: propidium iodide.

Chapter I

Introduction

Lung cancer is one of the most common malignancies worldwide and a leading cause of cancer-related deaths. It is increasing year by year in almost all areas of the world, except for a slight decrease in certain countries [1]. Lung cancer consists of heterogeneous groups in terms of pathological features and is generally classified into the following two major types, small cell lung carcinoma (SCLC) and non-small cell lung carcinoma (NSCLC). NSCLC also is a group of heterogeneous histological types, the majority of which are squamous cell carcinoma (SQC) and adenocarcinoma (ADC) with roughly similar frequencies (30-40% each), and large cell carcinoma (LCC) with a lower frequency (< 10%). SCLC comprises nearly 20% of lung cancer. ADC and LCC are further sub-classified into several categories, respectively. The classification of lung cancer is not only of academic interest but also of practical necessity, because the biological aggressiveness, responsiveness to therapeutic intervention and patients' prognosis are greatly different among the respective types [2].

Lung cancer originates from the airway epithelia of larger and smaller bronchi as well as of alveoli. While it is generally accepted that cancer cells are derived from progenitor or tissue stem cells, relatively little has been elucidated with regard to the identification of airway stem cells and the molecular mechanisms underlying their self-renewal and differentiation abilities [3-5], in contrast to other epithelial tissues such as the intestine, mammary gland, and skin [6].

The heterogeneity of lung cancer likely reflects differences in the site of origin (proximal versus peripheral), and, more importantly, in the type of cell of origin, i.e., progenitor (tissue stem) cells. The diversity of etiologic factors and target genes, the types of genetic insults, and the ensuing effects, activation or inactivation, on the genes involved, would also be responsible for the heterogeneity of lung cancer. In fact, tobacco smoke, containing more than 60 carcinogens, is generally accepted as the most important cause of almost all types of lung cancer, among which the genetic and molecular mechanisms of carcinogenesis differ considerably. The ensuing genetic alteration and epigenetic changes as well, could lead to dysfunction of molecular signal transduction pathways, which relate directly or indirectly to proliferation, differentiation, and death of the cell.

In our recent review article, we underscored that silencing alterations of both the *RB* and *TP53* genes are most likely to be important and early events in the development of SCLC, whereas alterations of the epidermal growth factor receptor (EGFR) signaling pathway, play significant and important roles in NSCLC carcinogenesis [7]. We also emphasized that alterations of both the *RB* and *TP53* genes are central to the carcinogenesis of SCLC, while many other factors including, achaete-scute complex homolog 1 (ASCL1) and thyroid transcription factor-1 (TTF-1), contribute to the development and biological behavior of SCLC [8].

The cancer stem cell (CSC) theory has proposed that a tumor cell subpopulation possessing self-renewal capacity, which forms only a small fraction of tumor tissue, is central in sustaining neoplastic lesions and is a potentially crucial target of cancer therapy [9-23]. The CSCs are possibly produced by either transformation of normal stem cells or multistep dedifferentiation of specialized progenitor cells through a progressive accumulation of genetic aberrations. Rapp, *et al.* [12] proposed a model of oncogene-induced plasticity for CSC origin by demonstrating reprogramming events triggered by a specific combination of oncogenes. Li, *et al.* [16] suggested that genomic instability is a driving force for transforming normal stem cells into CSCs and, in CSCs, a potential mechanism for cancer cell heterogeneity. The origin of CSCs and this mechanism are discussed in more detail in later other chapters [The publisher may modify this part].

The CSCs of lung cancers can be considered to originate from either airway stem cells, which have not been identified yet, or respective committed progenitor cells, such as bronchioloalveolar progenitor cells, basal/mucous secretory bronchial progenitor cells, and neuroendocrine progenitor cells (see the section: Origin of CSCs in Lung Cancers).

The CSC theory is tremendously attractive to both researchers and physicians, because the CSC is central to cancer cell biology and cancer therapy. The discovery of specific markers of CSCs, in the respective types of cancers, is particularly important. Furthermore, it is necessary to clarify the function of these molecules as the disruption of the signaling pathways and gene transcriptions that control the activity of CSCs is the final goal of CSC-targeting therapy. We emphasized that knowledge of CSC signaling pathways may lead to new treatment that kill or induce differentiation of CSCs and, could better contribute to cures [24]. These treatments could be designed to target CSCs in order to induce the differentiation of CSCs, or eliminate CSCs by inhibiting the maintenance of the stem-cell state. For instance, side population (SP) cells that are considered to represent CSCs (see below), of a human lung cancer cell line (A549) totally disappeared after treatment with the selective ATP-binding cassette transporter G2 (ABCG2) inhibitor fumitremorgin C [25]. As another example, a Hedgehog signaling inhibitor cyclopamine, strikingly reduced the *in vitro* invasive capacity of pancreatic cancer cell lines and also profoundly inhibited metastatic spread in an orthotopic xenograft model [26].

In regard to lung cancer, we also stressed the extreme importance of identifying specific CSC markers for the respective subtypes of lung cancer. SCLC and NSCLC (ADC, SQC, LCC, and others), for example, since they are quite different not only in phenotype but also in pathogenesis and biological behavior. In particular, SCLC is highly metastatic, drug-resistant, and rapidly fatal. The aggressiveness of SCLC may be attributable to an abundance of CSCs, as CSCs are drug-resistant and play a crucial role in cancer recurrence and metastasis. Alternatively, it is also possible that the CSCs of SCLC are endowed with specific biological properties, for instance, niche-independency or strong drug-resistance, or both. If SCLC-specific CSC markers were discovered, they would be extremely useful as targets of chemotherapy, for the establishment of therapeutic regimens, and for predictions of the prognosis, or outcome, of patients.

In this chapter book, we discuss the characteristics of normal airway stem/progenitor cells and CSCs in lung cancer by reviewing hitherto described study results. In addition, we demonstrate the potentially distinct differences in the mechanism of maintenance of CSCs between SCLC and NSCLC, primarily focusing upon aldehyde dehydrogenase (ALDH) based on our own experiments currently underway.

Chapter II

Stem Cells in Healthy and Injured Lung

Although the airway stem cell in a strict sense has not been identified yet, several lines of evidence support the existence of regional progenitors cells, such as bronchioloalveolar progenitor cells, basal/mucous secretory bronchial progenitor cells, and neuroendocrine progenitor cells, which maintain normal homeostasis as well as play roles in repair [3-5]. These progenitor cells expand their populations in response to various insults, including toxic substances, but do not become tumorigenic unless at least one genetic or epigenetic event occurs, for example instance, by tobacco smoke carcinogens [4,27].

Chapter III

Origin of CSCs in Lung Cancers

As in hematological malignancies and other solid cancers, the presence of subpopulations of cells endowed with CSC properties has been recognized in lung cancers. Like CSCs in other tissues, the CSCs of lung cancers can be considered to originate from either airway stem cells, which have not been identified yet, or respective committed progenitor cells, such as bronchioloalveolar progenitor cells, basal/mucous secretory bronchial progenitor cells, and neuroendocrine progenitor cells [3-5], resulting in the initiation of region-specific lung cancers [4].

Cell Markers for CSCs in Lung Cancers

CSC markers for lung cancer are a matter of some controversy, probably reflecting the tremendous heterogeneity of lung cancers in terms of cell of origin, etiology, pathology, biology, and molecular/genetic pathogenesis [2,7]. We herein briefly discuss these markers, paying special attention to the differences between SCLC and NSCLC; representative lung CSC markers reported to date are listed in Table 1.

Table 1. Cancer stem cell markers in SCLC and NSCLC

Category	Marker	SCLC	NSCLC
Cell surface marker	CD133	1. Eramo A, et al. [42] Cancer cells isolated from surgical specimens 2. Jiang T, et al. [52] H1688 cell line 3. Meng X, et al. [48] *H446 cell line	1. Eramo A, et al. [42] Cancer cells isolated from surgical specimens 2. Jiang T, et al. [52] H460, H125, H322, and H358 cell lines 3. Levina V, et al. [50] H460 cell line 4. Chen YC, et al. [51] Cancer cells isolated from surgical specimens 5. Meng X, et al. [48] *A549 cell line
	PODXL-1	1. Koch LK, et al. [69] Immunohistochemical analysis in surgical specimen tissue sections	
	uPAR	1. Gutova M, et al. [54] H1417, H69AR, H211, H1688, H1882, and H250 cell lines	

Table 1. (Continued)

Category	Maker	SCLC	NSCLC
Transporter	SP	1. Meng X, et al. [48] *H446 cell line	1. Ho MM, et al. [48] A549, H23, H460, HTB-58, H2170, and H441 cell lines 2. Meng X, et al. [48] *A549 cell line
	ABCG2		1. Sung JM, et al. [25] A549 cell line
Enzymatic activity	ALDH	1. Jiang T, et al. [52] Aldefluor assay in H1618 cell line 2. Moreb JS, et al. [93] RT-PCR, Western blotting, spectrophotometrical analysis and Aldefluor assay in SW210.5, H82, and SCLC-16HC cell lines	1. Ucar D, et al. [95] Spectrophotometrical analysis and Aldefluor assay in H522 cell line 2. Patel M, et al. [96]. Immunohistochemical analysis in surgical specimen tissue sections 3. Jiang F, et al. [49] Aldefluor assay in H460, H125, H322, and H358 cell lines 4. Moreb JS, et al. [93] RT-PCR, Western blotting, spectrophotometrical analysis and Aldefluor assay in A549, H522, H322, H157, H125, H460, H1299, LCLC-103H and ADLC-5M2H lung cancer cell lines, as well as Beas-2B non-cancerous airway cell line

Table 1.-(Continued)

Category	Marker	SCLC	NSCLC
Signaling pathway	Shh	1. Watkins DN, et al. [77] NCI-H1618, NCI-H60, NCI-H146, NCI-H209, NCI-H249, NCI-H82, and NCI-H417 cell lines 2. Yagui-Beltrán A, et al. [78] Review 3. Peacock CD, et al. [79] Review	1. Yagui-Beltrán A, et al. [78] Review 2. Peacock CD, et al. [79] Review
	Wnt/β-catenin	1. Yagui-Beltrán A, et al. [78] Review 2. Peacock CD, et al. [79] Review	1. Yagui-Beltrán A, et al. [78] Review 2. Peacock CD, et al. [79] Review 3. Levina V, et al. [50] H460 cell line

Category	Maker	SCLC	NSCLC
Transcription factor	Bmi1	1. Koch LK, et al. [69] Immunohistochemical analysis in surgical specimen tissue sections	1. Dovey JS, et al. [85] Bronchioloalveolar carcinoma (mouse)
	Oct-4		1. Levina V, et al. [50] H460 cell line 2. Chen YC, et al. [51] Cancer cells isolated from surgical specimens

SCLC: small cell lung carcinoma; NSCLC: non-small cell lung carcinoma; PODXL-1: podocalyxin-like protein 1; uPAR: urokinase plasminogen activator receptor; SP: side population; ABCG2: ATP binding cassette transporter superfamily member G2; ALDH: aldehyde dehydrogenase; Shh: Sonic hedgehog; Bmi1: B cell-specific Mo-MuLV integration site 1.*These authors reported that both of CD133+ and CD133- cells and of SP cells and non-SP cells exhibited the cancer initiating activity.The methods for analysis of ALDH activity and protein expression are specifically described, because the procedures employed may potentially lead to the differences in results, This table is modified from [24].

Chapter IV

CD133

CD133 was first reported as a novel marker for human hematopoietic stem and progenitor cells [28], and later found in some types of leukemic cells [29]. Prominin-1, which was identified on neuroepithelial stem cells in mice in 1997, is a mouse homolog of the human CD133 antigen [30]. The expression of CD133 has been detected in human central nervous system stem cells [31], human trophoblasts [32], human lymphatic/vascular endothelial precursor cells [33], and human prostatic epithelial stem cells [34]. The CD133 antigen is a 120kDa five-transmembrane domain glycoprotein, and its chromosomal location (4p16.2-p12) and amino acid sequence have been clarified [35]. Although its function is still unknown, CD133 may have a role in stem cell activation/maintenance, as shown by its coexpression with β1-integrin in the epidermal basal cells [36], release of CD133-carrying membrane particles into the extracellular space from neural progenitors and some epithelial cells [37], and potential regulatory activity of cell-cell contacts [38].

Recent studies have demonstrated that CD133 is a specific marker of CSCs in a wide spectrum of malignant tumors including brain tumors, colorectal cancers, pancreatic cancers, breast cancers, prostate cancers, ovarian cancers [39-41], and some lung cancers [42]. In contrast to the general consensus that CD133 is a ubiquitous CSC marker, several studies demonstrated that CD133-negative cells in certain human tumors also possess tumorigenic activity upon xenotransplantation into immunocompromised rodents [43-45]. These results imply that the CD133-negative subpopulation also contains cells with cancer initiating cell (CIC) activity. Mizrak, *et al.* [46] pointed out that CD133 is actually detected by its glycosylated epitope, AC133, and it is likely that AC133, but not CD133, is a more reliable CSC marker. Bidlingmaier, *et al.* [47] also suggested that the use of CD133 expression as a marker for CSC should be critically evaluated. These reports may explain the discrepancy observed in the results from different studies.

In regard to lung cancers, Eramo, *et al.* [42] reported that CD133 is a useful CSC marker in both SCLC and NSCLC. In contrast, Meng, *et al.* [48] reported more than 45% of A549 (NSCLC) and H446 (SCLC) cells to be CICs regardless of CD133 expression based on the results of cloning and tumorigenic analysis. Jiang, *et al.* [49] reported that, in NSCLC, cancer cells with strong ALDH activity (see below), showed CSC features and CD133 expression. Levina, *et al.* [50] demonstrated that NSCLC cells (H460) propagated a CD133-positive CSC-like cell population, in association with the expression of Oct-4 and high nuclear β-catenin (see below), after an *in vitro* treatment with anti-cancer drugs. Chen, *et al.* [51] reported that CD133-positive NSCLC cell lines display self-renewal and chemo-radio-resistant properties. Intriguingly, in SCLC, Jiang, *et al.* [52] demonstrated that achaete-scute complex homolog 1 (ASCL1) directly regulates ALDH1A1 and CD133 and that the $CD133^{high}$-$ALDH1A1^{high}$-$ASCL1^{high}$ subpopulation exhibits the features of CSCs both *in vitro* and *in vivo*. ASCL1 is a specific marker of SCLC and thought to play important roles in its phenotypic expression and biological aggressiveness [8,53].

Chapter V

Side Population

Hoechst 33342 dye-efflux side population (SP) bone marrow cells were first discovered as hematopoietic stem cells in mice [54]. Since then, SP cells with stem-cell-like capabilities have been found in a variety of human hematologic and solid malignancies. These cells show the features of CSCs characterized by self-renewal activity, differentiated progeny production, tumorigenicity, as well as the expression of CSC markers and stem cell genes [55]. Thus, SP cells can be assumed to be CSCs. Importantly, SP cells are highly resistant to chemotherapeutic agents and crucial in therapy resistance and tumor recurrence [55-57]. Zhou, *et al.* [58] showed that expression of the *ATP binding cassette transporter superfamily member G2* (*ABCG2*) gene is an important determinant of the SP phenotype, and that it might serve as a marker for stem cells from various sources. SP cells are usually isolated and purified by fluorescence activating cell sorting (FACS) using an ultraviolet (UV) laser. Recently, a new technique using a Violet-excited cell-permeable DNA-binding dye has been reported [59]. This method is inexpensive and yields the same results as UV-excited FACS [59]. In contrast, Wu, *et al.* [55] pointed out the following problems in using the SP phenotype as a CSC marker: 1) cells resistant to the Hoechst dye's toxicity do not consist only of stem-like cells, 2) variables in staining times, dye concentrations, and cellular concentrations can greatly affect the SP phenotype, and 3) cytometric gating strategies used to isolate SP cells lack the consistency of gating strategies used when staining with markers. These problems potentially lead to cross contamination of the SP and the non-SP fractions ultimately resulting in the production of confounding data. They emphasized that more stringent gating strategies are necessary and that a combination of isolation methods are required to enhance the purity of CSCs.

In lung cancers, Ho, *et al.* [60] reported that the SP cells in NSCLC cell lines were an enriched source of tumor-initiating cells with stem cell properties. Sung, *et al.* [25] suggested that ABCG2 played an important role in the multidrug resistance phenotype of SP cells in a NSCLC cell line, A549. In contrast, Meng, *et al.* [48] reported more than 45% of A549 (NSCLC) and H446 (SCLC) cells to be CICs, regardless of SP features based on the results of cloning and tumorigenic analyses.

Chapter VI

Aldehyde Dehydrogenase

The ALDH superfamily represents a divergently related group of enzymes that metabolize a wide variety of endogenous and exogenous aldehydes. In the human genome, at least 19 functional genes and 3 pseudogenes have been identified [61]. ALDH also contributes to the oxidation of retinol to retinoic acid, a modulator of cell proliferation, which may also modulate stem cell proliferation [62]. Murine and human hematopoietic stem cells [63-64], murine neural stem cells [65], normal and malignant human mammary stem cells [66], as well as normal and malignant human colorectal stem cells [62,67] exhibit ALDH activity and express this enzyme; strongly suggesting that strong ALDH activity and/or antigen expression can be used as a marker for stem cells in a variety of cancers. ALDH activity has been measured as substrate-oxidizing activity in whole cell lysate and the expression of the enzyme has been detected by immunoreactions with specific antibodies, such as Western blot and immunohistochemical analyses. Since the development of a new method using an ALDH-activated fluorescent substrate as a marker for the isolation of human hematopoietic stem cells [68], the so-called Aldefluor assay has been widely applied to the measurement and isolation of normal and malignant stem-cell-like cells in a variety of tissues [49,64-67]. This method is useful for isolating and purifying viable cells with high levels of ALDH activity for assays of the CSC properties of these cell populations.

Chapter VII

Other Lung CSC Markers

Koch, *et al.* [69] demonstrated that a majority of SCLC were immunohistochemically positive for the antibody against podocalyxin-like protein 1 (PODXL-1) and hypothesized that PODXL-1 is a potential CSC marker of SCLC. PODXL-1, belonging to a large family of cell surface sialomucins and being most closely related to CD34 and endoglycan [33,70,71], is expressed in primitive hematopoietic progenitors and thought to be a marker of embryonic and hematopoietic stem cells [72].

Gutova, *et al.* [73] found that SCLC cells positive for urokinase plasminogen activator receptor (uPAR) were resistant to traditional chemotherapies and speculated that they contain a putative CSC population. Urokinase plasminogen activator (uPA) and its receptor uPAR are instrumental in controlling membrane-associated extracellular proteolysis and transmembranous signaling, thus affecting cell migration and invasion [74]. uPAR is up-regulated by several oncogenic pathways including mutations of multiple oncogenes. Alfano, *et al.* [74] underlined the importance of uPAR signaling in the prevention of apoptosis.

Chapter VIII

Signaling Pathways in CSCs of Lung Cancers

Sonic Hedgehog

Sonic hedgehog (Shh) is expressed by the epithelial cells, and binds and signals to Patched1/2 receptors in the underlying mesenchyme [6,75,76].

Watkins, *et al.* [77] reported the significance of Hedgehog signaling in a subset of SCLCs. Yagui-Beltrán, *et al.* [78] and Peacock, *et al.* [79] reviewed the results of studies on CSC markers and signaling pathways in pulmonary carcinogenesis with special attention to the differences between SCLC and NSCLC. Both papers emphasized the potential importance of the Hedgehog and Wnt signaling pathways in SCLC and NSCLC (see below). Interestingly, human primary or immortalized bronchial epithelial cells exposed to cigarette smoke for only eight days in culture became tumorigenic in nude mice, in association with the activation of the Hedgehog and Wnt signaling pathways [80].

Wnt Signaling Pathway and Nuclear β-Catenin

For the maintenance and activation of normal stem cells, the Wnt/β-catenin signaling pathway is crucial, as distinctly demonstrated in the intestinal mucosa epithelia, epidermis, mammary gland [6], and other tissue [81]. The importance of Wnt signaling in cancer cells has been emphasized

[82], and the Wnt/β-catenin signaling cascade is a critical regulator not only of normal stem cells but also of CSCs [83]. Disruption of this signaling pathway at any step potentially causes disorders of stem cell activity and plays a crucial role in the development of cancer. For instance, sustained Wnt signaling mediated by the membrane receptor, Frizzled, stimulates the release of β-catenin from a cytoplasmic degradation complex composed of APC, Axin, GSK3-β and Dsh. This results in its movement into the nucleus and activation of Lef/Tcf transcription factors for c-Myc and cyclin D1 [82]. As another example, inactivation of APC due to a gene mutation also results in the release of β-catenin from the degradation complex, leading to the neoplastic transformation of colonic epithelial stem cells [11]. Thus, nuclear β-catenin is a hallmark for active Wnt signaling [75].

As described above, Yagui-Beltrán, *et al.* [87] and Peacock, *et al.* [79] emphasized the potential importance of the Wnt signaling pathway in SCLC and NSCLC in addition to the Hedgehog signaling pathway. Also as described above, human primary or immortalized bronchial epithelial cells exposed to cigarette smoke became tumorigenic in nude mice, being associated with the activation of not only the Hedgehog signaling pathway, but also the Wnt signaling pathway [80].

Chapter IX

Other Signaling Pathways and Transcription Factors in Lung CSCs

While the Wnt/β-catenin signaling pathway has been extensively investigated in many tissues including the lung, other signaling pathways are also important for controlling stem cell activity, including transmembranous Notch signaling and bone morphogenetic protein (BMP) signaling, mediated by the cell membrane receptor Bmpr1a [8,75]. However, we are only beginning to understand the roles these pathways play in CSC populations of lung cancers.

B cell-specific Mo-MuLV integration site 1 (Bmi1) is a member of the Polycomb group family of proteins and a downstream effector of the extracellular signaling molecule Shh. Bmi1 is implicated in the self-renewal of multiple stem cells including hematopoietic and neural stem cells [84]. Dovey, *et al.* [85] suggested that Bmi1 is critical for both normal and tumor bronchioloalveolar stem cell expansion in mice. Koch, *et al.* [69] demonstrated that a majority of SCLCs were immunohistochemically positive for antibodies against Bmi1. From these results, they hypothesized that Bmi1 is a potential CSC marker of SCLC.

Some studies suggest that Oct-4 is a potential CSC marker for lung cancers. Levina, *et al.* [50] demonstrated that a human large cell cancer cell line (H460) propagated a CSC-like cell population that showed CD133, Oct-4, and high nuclear β-catenin expression after an *in vitro* treatment with anti-cancer drugs. Chen, *et al.* [51] reported that Oct-4 expression plays a crucial role in maintaining the self-renewing, CSC-like, and chemo-radio-resistant properties of CD133-positive NSCLC cell lines. Oct-4 is a member of the POU transcription factor family known to be expressed in pluripotent stem cells and to function as a transcriptional regulator of multiple genes related to stemness [86].

In Vitro Assay

Several *in vitro* assays have been used to identify CSCs, including sphere-formation assays, serial colony-forming unit assays (re-plating assays), and label-retention assays [10,14]. Among them, sphere-formation assays are utilized in a wide range of tissue systems including lung cancers [42,87]. However, each of these methods has potential pitfalls that complicate interpretation of the results. For instance, difficulty in confirming clonality (single cell origin) has been pointed out [10]. In addition, the culture conditions used for these assays potentially exert selection pressures upon the cultured cells, resulting in the selection of only cell populations that are able to survive and proliferate under such specific conditions. The limitations of these *in vitro* assays should be kept in mind, and a combination of methods, including *in vivo* assays, is necessary for the identification and isolation of CSCs.

Chapter X

CSC Niche

The microenvironment surrounding normal and cancer stem cells, which provides the stem cell niche, plays multiple roles including as a mechanical anchorage for the stem cells and in cross-talk communication mediated by direct contact and/or indirect extracellular factors. For instance, Wnt ligands are produced and released from both stem cells and niche cells, BMP and Shh are released from niche cells and epithelial cells respectively, and Notch signaling is transmembranously transmitted between neighboring cells. The microenvironment may also provide signaling via the cell receptor integrin as suggested by its expression in prostatic CSCs [88] and its co-expression with AC133 (CD133) in the epidermal basal cells [36], as well as through metalloprotease-mediated lysophopholipid signaling [89].

The concept of a CSC niche is a matter of debate [90]. Two fundamental questions need to be answered: 1) Does a specific CSC niche exist? 2) If it does, what are the differences between the normal stem cell niche and CSC niche? Sneddon, *et al.* [23] removed some of the confusion regarding the CSC niche by proposing several possible models (Figure 1): 1) CSCs are capable of surviving in the normal stem cell niche, 2) a distinct CSC niche is necessary for activation, 3) CSCs may be capable of providing signals that instruct an otherwise quiescent niche to become activated, also known as "hijacking the niche", 4) CSCs could amplify an already existent activated niche, 5) CSCs may be niche-independent, that is, they themselves acquire the ability to maintain activity, and 6) there may be a discrete niche that is inhibitory for CSC maintenance. Accumulating evidence suggests that no single model fits all the diverse types of cancer. Further study is required to establish a universally acceptable CSC niche theory.

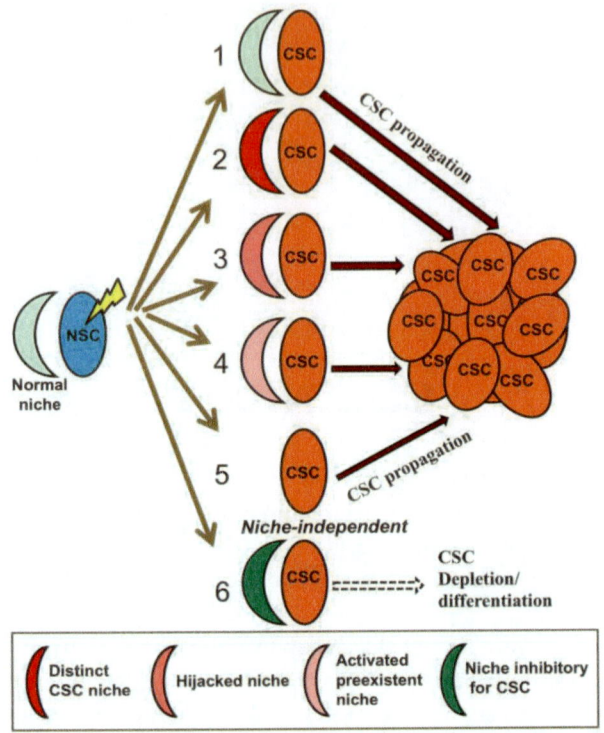

Modified from [24].

Figure 1. Hypothesis for the relationship between cancer stem cells (CSCs) and their niche. At least one genetic or epigenetic event (yellow arrow) is required to occur in a normal stem cell (NSC; or progenitor cell, not shown here) for a CSC initiation to develop (closed arrows). The CSCs may utilize the normal niche (1), require the distinct CSC niche (2), instruct an otherwise quiescent niche to become activated by providing signals ("hijacking the niche") (3), amplify an already existent activated niche (4), or become niche-independent (5). Furthermore, there may be a discrete niche that is inhibitory for CSC maintenance (6).

While the niche may also play an important role in the maintenance of CSCs from lung cancers, little has been elucidated yet. Hilbe, *et al.* [91] demonstrated by immunohistochemistry, a significant increase in CD133-positive vascular endothelial cells in patients with NSCLC and suggested an involvement of endothelial progenitor cells in the tumor vasculature and tumor growth, as well as possibly the maintenance and activation of CSCs. More studies of the lung CSC niche are required not only to understand the biological relationship between lung CSCs and their niche, but also for the development of therapeutic strategies for lung cancers.

Chapter XI

Brief Summary of Lung CSC Markers and Potential Problems

While investigations into the CSC markers of lung cancer are insufficient at this time, as discussed above and summarized in Table 1, we tentatively summarize the findings to date as follows: 1) CD133 expression and the SP phenotype are common CSC markers for SCLC and NSCLC. 2) The Wnt/β-catenin signaling pathway is also important in the maintenance and activation of CSCs in SCLC and NSCLC. 3) PODXL-1 and uPAR are potential CSC markers for SCLC, but their expression has not been well examined in NSCLC. 4) In regard to ALDH, results reported to date appear to be complicated. Its enzymatic activity has been demonstrated in SCLC and NSCLC cells by the Aldefluor assay, as well as by a spectrophotometrical assay [92-97]. On the other hand, an immunohistochemical analysis using antibodies against ALDH1A1 and ALDH3A1 in tissue sections of surgical specimens of lung cancer, demonstrated the expression of these ALDH isozymes in NSCLC cases, but not in SCLC cases, suggesting that the ALDH protein expression was limited to CSCs in NSCLC [96]. In contrast, Moreb, *et al.* [93] reported that in their studies using several SCLC and NSCLC cell lines there were good correlations between the results of a Western blot analysis, a spectrophotometrical analysis, and the Aldefluor assay, in spite of a few exceptions (see below). The discrepancy among these results may be attributable to the difference in the antibodies used and the difference between the *in vitro* and *in vivo* conditions as well.

Though evidence is still poor, it is supposed that distinct differences in the mechanism of ALDH expression and activity, as well as the role of ALDH in the maintenance/activation of CSCs, exist between SCLC and NSCLC. Furthermore, the exact mechanism and role of ALDH in the maintenance of the stemness of normal stem cells and CSCs are still unknown. To try to resolve these issues, we have carried out investigations which are described in the following section.

Recent Findings in ALDH and CSC of the Lung

As described above, ALDH activity and its protein expression have been reported to be useful normal stem cell and CSC markers in a wide range of tissues [66,92,96-98]. These ALDHs play pluripotent roles in endobiotic and xenobiotic metabolism through specific metabolic pathways. One important issue to be addressed is which ALDH isozymes are responsible for the ALDH activity used to identify stem cell progenitors. Several studies have demonstrated that ALDH activity is needed for the differentiation of primitive progenitors into mature cells, thus fulfilling one of the defining characteristics of multipotent stem cells, and some lines of evidence suggest that ALDH1A1 is an important marker of hematopoietic stem cell progenitors [92]. In fact, ALDH1A1 is one of the enzymes involved in the production of retinoic acid from retinol, and retinoic acid is considered significantly important in maintaining a balance between hematopoietic stem cell self-renewal and differentiation [92].

Moreb, *et al.* [93] systemically evaluated ALDH expression in several lung cancer cell lines (SCLC and NSCLC cell lines), utilizing the Aldefluor assay, a Western blotting, and a spectrophotometry and found a very good correlation between the results of all three. They concluded that the Aldefluor assay can be adapted successfully to measure ALDH activity in lung cancer cells, providing real time changes in ALDH activity in viable cells treated with chemotherapy or siRNA. They emphasized the importance of the use of mixed populations of cells with high ALDH levels and cells lacking ALDH activity when ALDH activity is measured by the Aldefluor assay in cells known to have high ALDH levels. Importantly, they carried out double Aldefluor and propidium iodide (PI) staining to delineate dead cells. According to their results, while ALDH expression levels were heterogeneous among the cell lines examined, overall findings revealed low levels of ALDH activity in SCLC cell lines, while higher levels were detected in some, but not all, NSCLC cell lines. The results correlated very well with protein and enzymatic activity as measured by the Western blot analysis and the spectrophotometrical assay, respectively. Intriguingly, there was one exception: The SW210.5 (SCLC) cell line registered only a small amount of ALDH activity in the spectrophotometrical assay and expressed only small amounts of ALDH1A1 and ALDH3A1 proteins in the Western blot analysis, whereas the Aldefluor assay showed high levels of ALDH activity (50% of the cells). This SCLC cell line (SW210.5) was shown to express mRNA for ALDH1A1 and ALDH2, but not ALDH3A1, by the semi-quantitative reverse transcription polymerase chain reaction (RT-PCR) assay.

Our preliminary experiments revealed very high levels of ALDH1A1 mRNA expression in some SCLC and NSCLC cell lines. We also observed considerable discrepancies between mRNA levels detected by the quantitative RT-PCR assay, protein levels analyzed by Western blotting, and the proportion of cells with enzymatic activity measured by the Aldefluor assay in several SCLC and NSCLC cell lines.

Aiming to elucidate the mechanism underlying the discrepancies observed in preliminary experiments and the previous study, we carried out the following experiments.

Chapter XII

ALDH mRNA Expression - Its Correlation with the most Common CSC Marker CD133

The quantitative RT-PCR assay revealed that ALDH1A1 mRNA was expressed at detectable levels in seven out of nine SCLC cell lines (77.8%), three of which expressed it at unequivocally high levels (33.3%), while it was expressed in four of the 18 NSCLC cell lines, two of which expressed it at high levels (11.1%)(Figure 2). On the other hand, ALDH2 was expressed in eight of the nine SCLC cell lines and 17 of the 18 NSCLC cell lines. The levels were lower on the whole than those of ALDH1A1 and did not remarkably differ among the cell lines. mRNA of CD133, the most commonly used CSC marker, was expressed only in SCLC cell lines (66.7%, or six out of nine cell lines), and its level in SCLC cell lines tended to be associated with the level of ALDH1A1, but not ALDH2. The findings suggested ALDH1A1 to have an important significance in the maintenance of stemness in lung cancer cells, and might account for the highly malignant activity of SCLCs.

ALDH Protein Expression in Lung Cancer Cell Lines

ALDH protein was detected by Western blotting using a non-selective antibody, which binds both ALDH1A1 and ALDH2 proteins (clone 44, BD transduction, Palo Alto, CA).

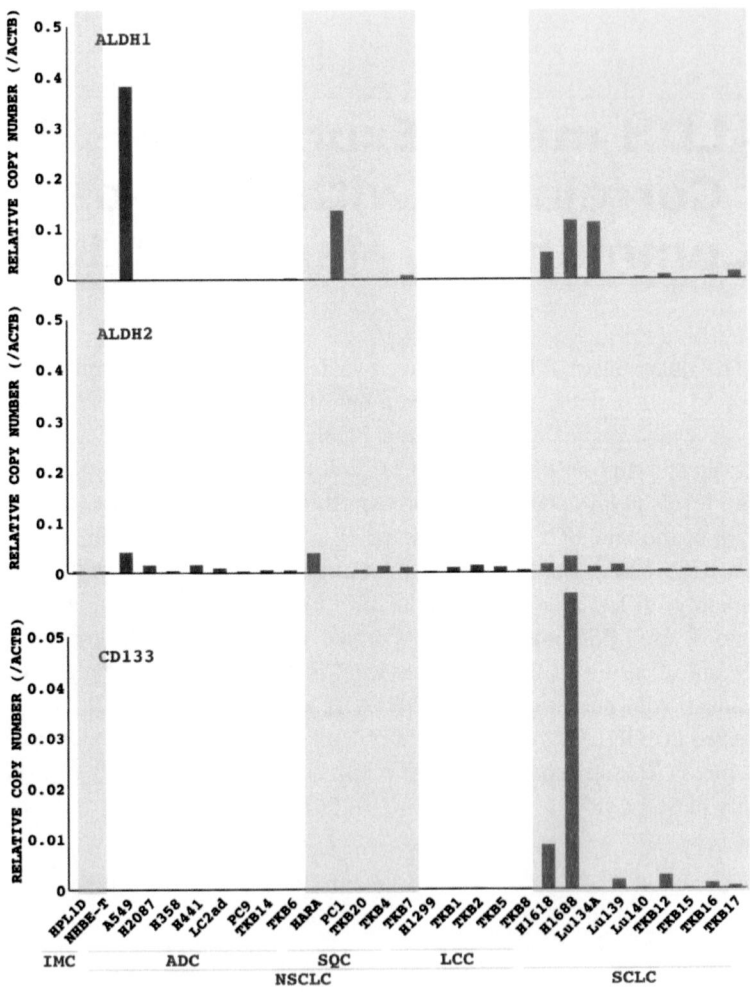

Figure 2. Expression of ALDH1, ALDH2 and CD133 mRNA in immortalized human airway cell and lung cancer cell lines. Levels of mRNA of ALDH1, ALDH2 and

CD133 and β-actin (ACTB) were measured by quantitative RT-PCR. The mRNA levels of ALDH1 (upper panel), ALDH2 (second panel) and CD133 (lower panel) relative to that of ACTB in immortalized human airway cells and lung cancer cells are presented. IMC, immortalized human airway cell lines; ADC, adenocarcinoma cell lines; SQC, squamous cell carcinoma cell lines; LCC, large cell carcinoma cell lines; NSCLC, non-small cell lung carcinoma cell lines; SCLC, small cell lung carcinoma cell lines. The experimental materials and methods are as follows. An immortalized human airway epithelial cell line (16HBE14o, Simian virus 40 (SV40)-transformed human bronchial epithelial cells) described by Cozens AL, *et al.* [102] was kindly provided by Gruenert DC (California Pacific Medical Center Research Institute, CA) via Kaneko T (Division of Respiratory Disease Center, Yokohama City Medical Center Hospital, Yokohama, Japan). A sub-clone of 16HBE14o cells, described as NHBE-T in this book, was used. An immortalized airway epithelial cell line (HPL1D, SV40-transformed human small airway epithelial cells) established by Masuda A, *et al.* [103], was provided by Takahashi T (Division of Molecular Carcinogenesis, Center for Neurological Disease and Cancer, Nagoya University Graduate School of Medicine, Nagoya, Japan). Human lung cancer cell lines (A549, H358, H2087, H1618, H1688 and H1299) were purchased from American Type Culture Collection (ATCC, Manassas, VA). Human lung cancer cell lines, LC2/ad, Lu134A and Lu140 were obtained form Riken Cell Bank (Tsukuba, Japan), and PC9, PC1 and HARA from Immuno-Biological Laboratories Co. (Gunma, Japan). Human lung cancer cell lines, TKB1, TKB2, TKB4, TKB5, TKB6, TKB7, TKB8, TKB12, TKB15, TKB16, TKB17 and TKB20, were kindly provided by Kamma H (Department of Pathology, Kyorin University School of Medicine, Tokyo, Japan) via Yazawa T (Department of Pathology, Yokohama City University School of Medicine, Yokohama Japan). The cells were cultured and grown in DEMEM (Sigma Aldrich, St. Louis, MO) (NHBE-T, HPL1D, A549, H358, H2087, PC9, PC1, HARA, LC2/ad, TKB1, TKB2, TKB4, TKB5, TKB6, TKB7, TKB8, TKB20 and H1299) or RPMI1640 medium (Sigma) (H1618, H1688, Lu130, Lu134A, Lu140, TKB12, TKB15, TKB16 and TKB17) supplemented with 10% heat-inactivated fetal bovine serum (FBS) (Sigma), 100 units/ml of penicillin (Sigma), and 100 μg/ml of streptomycin (Sigma). Total RNA was extracted from the cells with Isogen reagents (NIPPON GENE, Tokyo, Japan). First-strand cDNA was synthesized from total RNA using the SuperScript First-Strand Synthesis System according to the protocols of the manufacturer (Invitrogen, Carlsbad, CA). The cDNA generated was used as a template in real-time PCR with SYBR Premix EXTaq (Takara, Kyoto, Japan). The primer set used for ALDH1A1 was forward (F), 5'- agtgcccctttggtggattc; reverse (R), 5'- aagagcttctctccactcttg. That for ALDH2 was, F, 5'- ctacacacgccatgaacctg; R, 5'- caaccacgtttccagttg. That for CD133 was, F, 5'- ttgtggcaaatcaccaggta; R, 5'- gatgttgggtctcagtcggt. That for ACTB was, F, 5'-tggcacccagcacaatgaa; R, 5'- ctaagtcatagtccgcctagaagca. The mean of the copy number of ALDH1A1, ALDH2 or CD133 normalized to the value for ACTB mRNA was obtained from triplicate reactions.

The protein was expressed at high levels in two of the nine SCLC cell lines (22.2%), and two of the 18 NSCLC cell lines (11.1%)(Figure 3). The level of protein paralleled well the level of ALDH1A1 mRNA, but not ALDH2 mRNA, in NSCLC cell lines, suggesting that the protein detected by the

Western blot analysis was ALDH1A1 rather than ALDH2 (Figure 2 and Figure 3). Thus, we describe the protein detected here by the Western blot analysis as ALDH1A1. Interestingly, one SCLC cell line (Lu134) with a high level of ALDH1A1 mRNA did not express ALDH1A1 (either ALDH1A1 or ALDH2) (Figure 2). This result is similar to a previous observation that a SCLC cell line, SW210.5, expressed ALDH1 mRNA, but only a very small amount of protein [93]. These findings suggest a potential post-translational mechanism to be involved in ALDH1A1 protein expression in some SCLC cells.

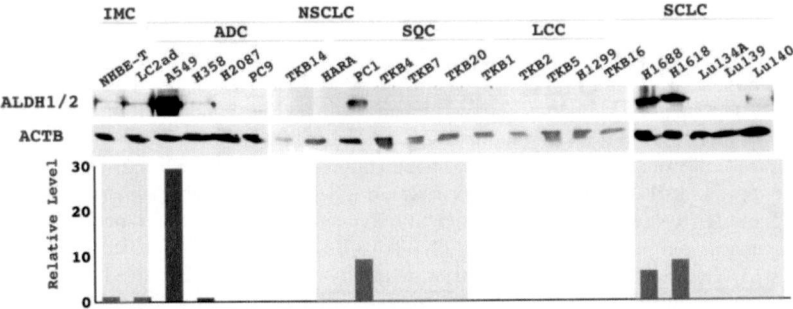

Figure 3. Expression of ALDH1A1/ALDH2 (ALDH1/2) protein in lung cancer cell lines. ALDH1/2 (top panel) and β-actin (ACTB) (second panel) protein expressions were analyzed by Western blotting. Levels of ALDH1/2 and ACTB protein were semi-quantified with a densitometer (NIH Image; National Institute of Mental Health at Bethesda, MD). The level of ALDH1/2 normalized to that of ACTB is presented in a graph (third panel). IMC, immortalized human airway epithelial cell lines; ADC, adenocarcinoma cell lines; SQC, squamous cell carcinoma cell lines; LCC, large cell carcinoma cell lines; NSCLC, non-small cell lung carcinoma cell lines; SCLC, small cell lung carcinoma cell lines. The experimental materials and methods are as follows. The cell lines (the details of the experimental materials are described in the legend for Figure 2) grown to sub-confluence were solved with extraction buffer, as described elsewhere [104]. After centrifugation, supernatants were recovered as protein extracts. The extracts were mixed with equal volumes of 2×sample buffer [104], and then boiled. The samples were subjected to sodium dodecyl sulfate-polyacrylamide gel electrophoresis, and transferred onto PVDF membranes (Amersham, Arlington Heights, IL). The membranes were incubated with nonfat dry milk in 0.01 M Tris-buffered saline containing 0.1% Tween-20 (TBS-T) to block non-immunospecific protein binding, and then with 0.1 µg/ml of a primary antibody which non-selectively binds to both ALDH1A1 and ALDH2 (clone 44, BD Transduction, San Jones, CA) or a primary antibody against ACTB (Sigma). After washing with TBS-T, the membranes were incubated with animal-matched horseradish peroxidase-conjugated secondary antibodies (Amersham). Immunoreactivity was visualized with the enhanced chemiluminescence system (ECL, Amersham).

Chapter XIII

ALDH Activity in Lung Cancer Cell Lines

The fraction of cells with ALDH activity was measured with the Aldefluor assay. The two SCLC cell lines with high ALDH1A1 protein levels (H1688 and H1618) had fractions of cells with strong ALDH activity (Figure 4). All of the SCLC cell lines with very weak ALDH protein expression (the faint bands detected by Western blotting in these cell lines were presumably ALDH2, because these cell lines expressed only ALDH2, not ALDH1A1, mRNA) had only a small fraction (less than 10%) of cells with ALDH activity. On the other hand, among NSCLC cell lines examined (A549, PC1, H441, H2087 and H1299) (not all data shown), only one (PC1) had fraction of cells with strong ALDH activity (Figure 4). One cell line, with high ALDH1A1 protein levels (A549), unexpectedly had only a very small fraction of cells with strong ALDH activity. Summarizing the findings, ALDH1A1 protein expression was closely associated with ALDH activity in SCLC cells, but not necessarily in NSCLC cells; suggesting the potential post-translational mechanism to be involved in activation of ALDH1A1 protein in NSCLCs.

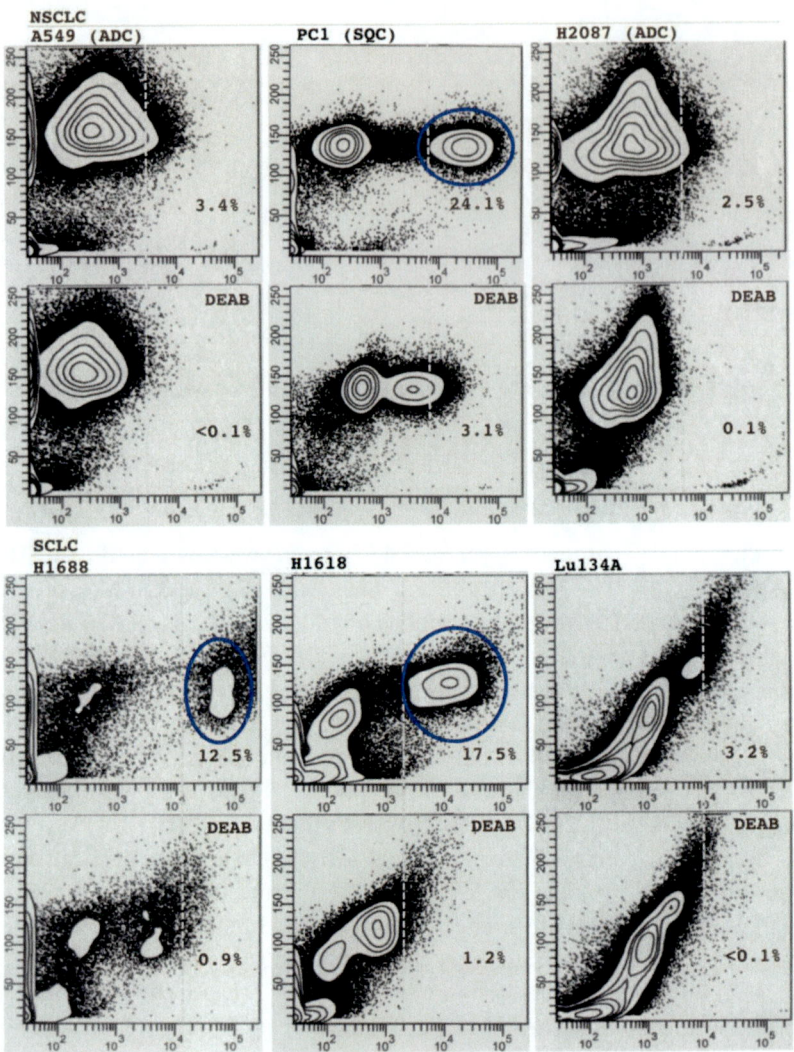

Figure 4. Measurement of fraction of cells with ALDH activity (Aldefluor assay) in lung cancer cell lines. Cells were labeled with Aldefluor (BODIPY-aminoacetaldehyde [BAAA]) (Stem cell technology Inc., Vancouver, Canada) with or without the ALDH inhibitor diethylaminobenzaldehyde (DEAB) (Stem cell technology). The proportion of fraction of cells with ALDH activity was measured by flow cytometer. The X-axis is fluorescence intensity (log scale), and the Y-axis is forward scatter level (linear scale). The fraction of cells with strong ALDH activity is shown (blue circle). NSCLC, non-small cell lung carcinoma cell lines; ADC, adenocarcinoma cell lines; SQC, squamous cell carcinoma cell lines; SCLC, small

cell lung carcinoma cell lines. The experimental materials and methods are as follows. The details of the cell lines examined are described in the legend for Figure 1. Cells with ALDH activity was labeled using Aldefluor assay kit (Stem cell technology) according to the manufacturer's instructions. Briefly, 1.0×10^6 cells in 1 ml of Aldefluor assay buffer with BAAA at a concentration of 1.5 mM were incubated for 45 min at 37C. In each experiment, a sample of cells was treated under identical conditions with 50 mM of a specific ALDH inhibitor (DEAB) to serve as a negative control. The fraction of cells with ALDH activity labeled by Aldefluor was measured with a flow cytometer (BD Science, San Jose, CA) (excitation wave length 488 nm and emission wave length 525 nm (green fluorescence)). Data for 1.0×10^5 cells were collected.

Chapter XIV

Primary Structure of ALDH1A1 mRNA

To elucidate the possible involvement of a mutation (or polymorphism) or splicing disorder in the difference among the levels of mRNA, protein and activity, which was observed in Lu134 SCLC and A549 NSCLC cells, the nucleotide sequence of open reading frames of cDNA were analyzed. No mutation (or polymorphism) causing an amino acid substitution was found in either cell line (data not shown). However, interestingly, short mRNA variant (258 base pairs in the open reading frame, encoding 86 amino acids: see Figure 5) was found in the Lu134A cell line. This variant was found in three of eight sub-clones (37.5%) in our sub-cloning experiment (part of the result is shown in Figure 5). The result suggested the possible involvement of such a variant in the post-transcriptional regulation of ALHD1A1 expression, and also implied a potential difference between SCLC and NSCLC, although further screening of a larger number of cell lines and primary lung cancers is required to test this idea.

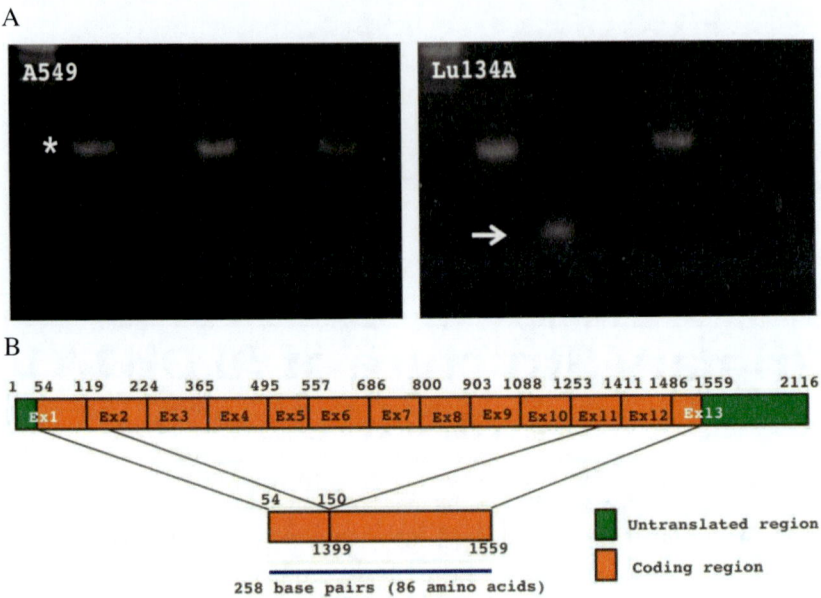

Figure 5. Analysis of primary structure of mRNA of ALDH1A1. The protein-coding sequence in ALDH1A1 mRNA was amplified by RT-PCR using primers, forward, 5'-aggagccgaatcagaaatgtc; reverse, 5'-aagagcttctctccactcttg, according to the method descried in the legend for Figure 2. The PCR product was sub-cloned into the plasmid vector pT7Blue (Novagen, Darmstadt, Germany), and then its size was checked by PCR using universal primers (T7 promoter primer and M13M4 primer (Novagen)). (A) A representative result from A549 (ADC) and Lu134A (SCLC) cells is shown. Shorter PCR products (faster migrating band (arrow)) were found in some sub-clones from Lu134A. Bands of expected size with a full-length coding region of ALDH1A1 (NCBI accession # NM_000689) are indicated with an asterisk. (B) Schema of the primary structure of the consensus mRNA and the shorter variant with their mRNA spliced sites in the ALDH1A1 gene, is shown. The shorter novel variant consists of parts of exon 1, exon2, exon 11, exon 12, and exon 13. "Ex" in figure means exon.

Chapter XV

Post-translational Modification of ALDH1A1 Protein

Since no mutation was found in the cell line with the lag between ALDH1/2 protein expression and ALDH activity (A549 cells), we next verified the possible involvement of a post-translational modification. To screen for such a modification, two-dimensional Western blot analysis was performed with A549 (NSCLC) and H1688 (SCLC) cells (Figure 6). While the results did not reveal unequivocal evidence of a modification, the ALDH1A1 protein migrated slightly faster in A549 cells (Figure 6). To elucidate the mechanism underlying the lag between ALDH1A1 protein expression and ALDH activity, further investigations of protein structure and modifications such as glycosylation, phosphorylation and acetylation status, are required.

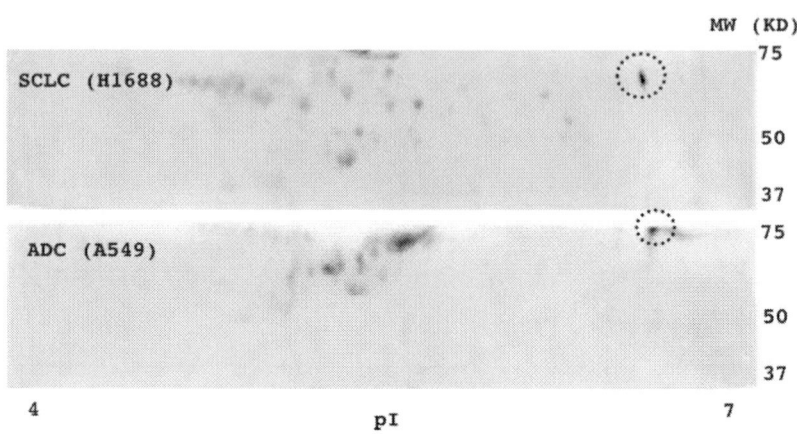

Figure 6. Two-dimensional Western blotting analysis of ALDH1A1/ALDH2 (ALDH1/2) protein in small cell lung carcinoma (SCLC) cell line (top panel; H1688) and an adenocarcinoma (ADC) cell line (bottom panel; A549) and. Spots of ALDH1 /2 protein were circulated with dashed lines. MW, molecular weight; KD, kilo-dalton; pI, isoelectric point plugin. The experimental materials and methods are as follows. Two-dimensional electrophoresis (2-DE) was carried out using a horizontal electrophoresis system (Maltiphor II; Amersham) according to the manufacture's instruction. Briefly, equal amount of protein sample was subjected to the first-dimensional isoelectric focusing, and followed by the second dimensional sodium dodecyl sulfate-polyacrylamide gel electrophoresis. The details of method are described elsewhere [105,106]. The separated proteins on the 2-DE gels were transferred onto a polyvinylidene difluoride membrane (FluoroTrans® PVDF Membrane, Nippon Genetics, Tokyo, Japan). The membranes were incubated with nonfat dry milk in 0.01 M Tris-buffered saline containing 0.1% Tween-20 (TBS-T) to block non-immunospecific protein binding, and then with 0.1 µg/ml of a primary antibody, which non-selectively binds to both ALDH1A1 and ALDH2 (clone 44, BD Transduction). After washing with TBS-T, the membranes were incubated with animal-matched horseradish peroxidase-conjugated secondary antibodies (Amersham). Immunoreactivity was visualized with the enhanced chemiluminescence system (ECL, Amersham).

(data not shown), supporting our supposition. Furthermore ALDH1/2 protein expression tended to decrease in parallel with the dedifferentiation process, as a large proportion of poorly differentiated NSCLCs expressed the protein only faintly (data not shown). In well-differentiated and *in situ* NSCLCs, ALDH1/2 expression may still be regulated by the physiological system (it may be lost during progression process to develop poorly differentiated ones). Although further investigation is required to elucidate the mechanism and significance of such a downregulation of ALDH1/2 protein expression in primary lung cancers, the results obtained here imply that ALDH1/2 protein plays diverse roles in different situations, and is not a universal stem cell marker. The mechanism to induce ALDH1/2 protein expression and its significance are likely to differ among the non-cancerous airway epithelia, NSCLCs and SCLCs.

A

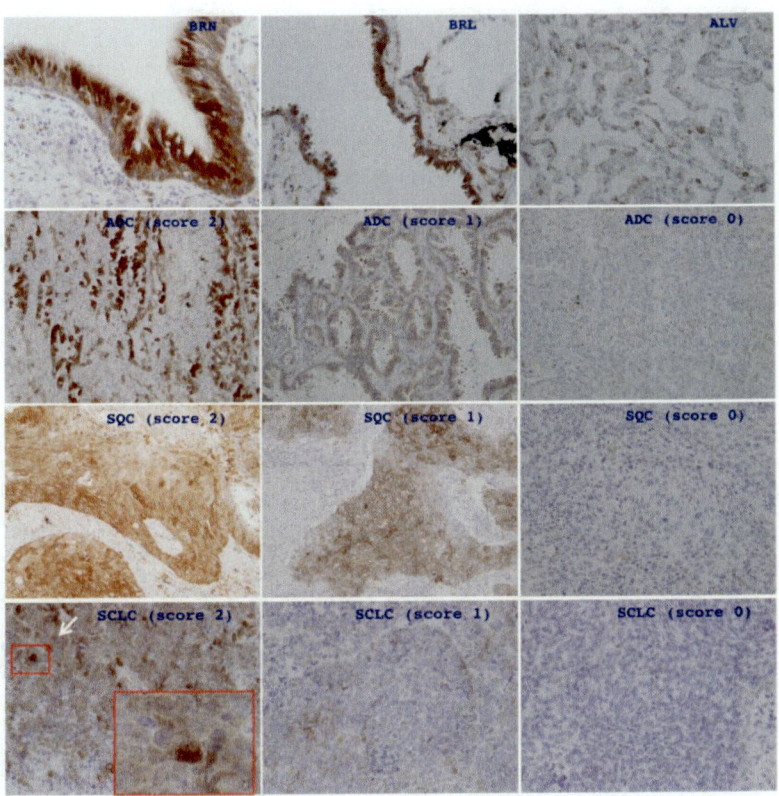

Chapter XVI

ALDH Protein Expression in Primary Lung Cancers

ALDH protein expression in primary lung tumors was examined by immunohistochemistry using a non-selective antibody, which binds both ALDH1A1 and ALHD2 proteins (ALDH1/2). The protein expression was detected in three of nine SCLCs (33.3%) and in 41 of 70 NSCLCs (58.6%)(Table 2). The levels tended to be higher in NSCLC, especially SQC, than in SCLC (Figure 5). The results were similar to those reported by Patel, *et al.* [96], who found in their immunohistochemical analysis that the ALDH isozymes 1A1 and 1A3 were expressed at significantly higher levels in NSCLC than in SCLC [96]. However, we have found that there is a discrepancy between the results of Western blotting for cancer cell lines and immunohistochemistry for primary lung cancers. The frequency of ALDH1/2 protein expression was considerably higher in primary cancers than in cell lines among NSCLCs, whereas it was similar between the two among SCLCs (Figure 3 and Table 2). Moreover, non-cancerous airway cells *in vivo*, i.e., both the bronchial, bronchiole and alveolar epithelial cells, exhibited high levels of immunohistochemical expression of ALHD1/2 protein compared to cancer cells in all cases examined (Figure 7 and Table 2). Interestingly, the two non-cancerous immortalized airway epithelial cell lines (NHBE-T and HPL1D) showed very weak expression of ALDH1/2 protein *in vitro*. The ALDH family is expressed in response to toxic stress [99-101]. The marked expression of ALDH1/2 protein in non-cancerous airway epithelial cells *in vivo* is supposed to be induced by external stimuli such as dust, cigarette smoke and so on. In NSCLCs, ALDH1/2 protein tended to be expressed more strongly among *in situ* parts than invasive parts

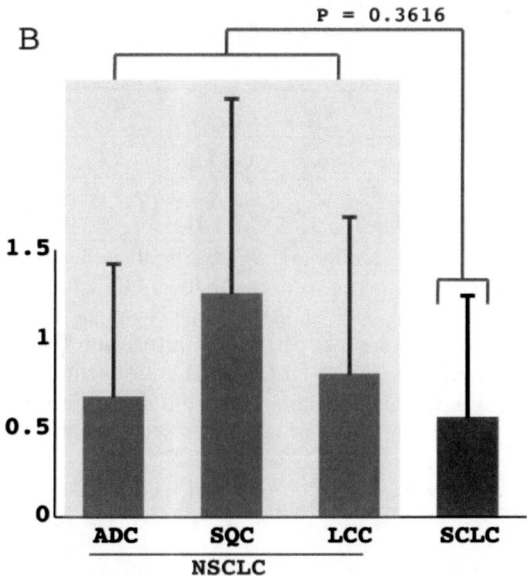

Figure 7. Expression of ALDH1A1/ALDH2 (ALDH1/2) protein in non-cancerous airway epithelia and primary lung cancers. (A) Representative photographs of immunohistochemistry of surgical specimens of non-cancerous airway epithelia (top panels) and lung cancers (the other panels) are shown. Magnifications are ×200 in, non-cancerous airway epithelia (bronchus, bronchiole and alveolus), adenocarcinoma (ADC), squamous cell carcinoma (SQC) and small cell lung carcinoma (SCLC), and ×400 in the inset of SCLC. Levels of ALDH1/2 expression were evaluated according to a scoring system; negative (score 0), unequivocally strong (score 2), and positive but weaker than a score of 2 (score 1). (B) Seventy-nine tumors (49 ADCs, 16 SQCs, 5 large cell carcinomas, and 9 SCLCs) were examined. The mean and standard deviation (error bar) among each histological type are shown in graph. Differences were analyzed with Student's t-test, and P value is indicated. The experimental materials and methods are as follows. All cases examined were of lung cancer patients who underwent surgical resection at the Kanagawa Prefectural Cardiovascular and Respiratory Disease Center Hospital (Yokohama, Japan) between 2001 and 2008. Informed consent for research use was obtained from all the subjects providing materials. Tissue sections (4 μm thick), cut from the formalin-fixed and paraffin-embedded tissue block with largest tumor dimension, were deparaffinized and rehydrated, and incubated with 3% hydrogen peroxide to block endogenous peroxidase activities. The sections were incubated with 5% goat serum to block non-immunospecific protein binding. After antigen retrieval treatment, boiling in citrated buffer (0.01 M, pH6.0) to restore the masked epitope, the sections were incubated with a primary antibody, which non-selectively binds to both ALDH1A1 and ALDH2 (clone 44, BD Transduction). Immunoreactivity was visualized with an Envision detection system (DAKOcytomation, Carpinteria, CA), and the nuclei were counterstained with hematoxylin.

Table 2. Positive rate of immunohistochemical expression of ALDH1/2 in NSCLC and SCLC

	NSCLC			SCLC
[Number of cases]	ADC [49]	SQC [16]	LCC [5]	[9]
Positive rate % [No.]	51.0% [25]	87.5% [14]	40.0% [2]	33.3% [3]

NSCLC, non-small cell lung carcinoma; SCLC, small cell lung carcinoma; ADC, adenocarcinoma; SQC, squamous cell carcinoma; LCC, large cell carcinoma; Chi-square test (among all, $P = 0.0254$; NSCLC versus SCLC, $P = 0.154$) Immunohistochemical analysis was performed in formalin-fixed tumor sections using a primary antibody against ALDH (BD transduction, Palo Alto, CA). Immunoreactivity was visualized with an Envision detection system (DAKO). If 5% or more of neoplastic cells in a tumor showed immunohistochemical expression of ALDH, it was judged as positive.

Chapter XVII

Conclusion

As is widely accepted, among lung cancers, SCLC and NSCLC are distinctly different in terms of biological behavior and pathogenesis. We have hypothesized that the CSCs of these two major subtypes of lung cancer possess different biological properties and that the abundance of CSCs population differs between the two. We have here focused upon ALDH to confirm such a potential difference.

The proportion of cells with strong ALDH activity tended to be associated with the CD133 mRNA level, especially in SCLC cell lines (Figure 2). Recently, Jiang, *et al.* [52] demonstrated in SCLC cell lines, that the ALDH1A1^{high}-CD133^{high}-ASCL1^{high} subpopulation exhibits the features of CSCs and that ASCL1 directly regulates ALDH1A1 and CD133 both *in vitro* and *in vivo*. Previous observations [60] are consistent with our results and also support the hypothesis that the size of the CSC fraction (population) could be one of the causes of highly malignant activity of SCLC. Importantly, however, not all SCLCs among cell lines and primary tumors were found to have either protein expression or a fraction of cells with high ALDH activity (Figure 4, Figure 7 and Table 2). We thus speculate that the ALDH activity is only one of the factors determining the stemness of CSCs in SCLCs. Alternatively, ALDH1A1 protein expression or ALDH activity is just part of the machinery to maintain stemness and might have significance only in some fractions of SCLCs. On the other hand, Ucar, *et al.* [95] proposed ALDH activity to be a CSC marker in a NSCLC cell line (NIH-H522 LCC cell line). Moreover, Jiang, *et al.* [49] reported that, in NSCLCs, cancer cells with strong ALDH1A1 activity, which were isolated using the Aldefluor assay followed by fluorescence-activated cell sorting, showed CSC features and CD133 expression. They proposed that ALDH1A1 is a lung cancer stem cell-associated marker, being a potential prognostic factor and therapeutic target for the treatment of patients with lung cancer. In our experiments, one NSCLC cell line (PC1 [SQC]) had a high ALDH1A1 protein level and a large fraction of cells with strong ALDH activity (Figure 3 and Figure 5), but did not express CD133 mRNA. Taken together, it is supposed that there is considerable heterogeneity in the mechanism maintaining the stemness of CSCs of SCLCs and NSCLCs.

Aside from the maintenance of stemness, another interesting finding of our experiments was that the level of ALDH1A1 mRNA did not always parallel the level of protein in SCLC cell lines, whereas, in NSCLC cell lines (Figure 3 and Figure 4) the level of protein was not always consistent with that of activity. Furthermore, the *in vivo* findings revealed that either non-cancerous airway epithelia or low-grade neoplasms such as well-differentiated, or *in situ,* NSCLCs showed stronger immunohistochemical expression of ALDH1A1 (possibly ALDH2 too) protein than less-differentiated cancer cells.

From the current findings, the mechanism and pathway which regulate the expression of ALDH1A1 mRNA and its protein, as well as its enzymatic activity and its role vary in different situations and among non-cancerous airway cells, NSCLCs and SCLCs, as well as among individual tumors. We speculate that ALDH1A1, its expression and/or activity, is only one of the factors determining the stemness in lung cancers.

In conclusion, the CSCs in SCLC and NSCLC differ distinctly from each other in terms not only of their abundance (suggested by CD133 mRNA levels) but also of the regulatory mechanism of ALDH1A1 expression and its activity, as well as its role in the maintenance/activation of stemness. The investigation of the mechanism of ALDH activation and its role in the maintenance of the stemness, not only of CSCs but also of normal stem cells, would provide a novel paradigm for stem cell biology and the development of a molecular targeting therapy for lung cancer.

Acknowledgments

This work was supported by the Japanese Ministry of Education, Culture, Sports, and Science (Tokyo Japan), Smoking Research Foundation (Tokyo, Japan), and by a grant from Yokohama Medical Facility (Yokohama, Japan). We especially thank Hideaki Mitsui (Department of Pathology, Yokohama City University Graduate School of Medicine, Yokohama, Japan), Shigeko Iwanade (Division of Pathology, Kanagawa Prefectural Cardiovascular and Respiratory Center Hospital, Yokohama, Japan), and Tetsukan Woo (Department of General Thoracic Surgery, Kanagawa Prefectural Cardiovascular and Respiratory Center Hospital, Yokohama, Japan) for assistance.

References

[1] Parkin, M., Tyczynski, JE., Boffetta, P., Samet, J., Shields, P., Caporaso, N. Lung cancer epidemiology and etiology. In: Travis, W.D., Brambilla, E., Muller-Hermelink, H.K., Harris, C.C. (eds). *Tumours of the lung. Tumours of the lung, pleura, thymus and heart. World Health Organization Classification of Tumours. Pathology and Genetics.* Lyon, IARC Press 2004; 12-15.

[2] Travis, W.D., Brambilla, E., Muller-Hermelink, H.K., Harris, C.C. (eds). IARC Press: Lyon, 2004; 9-124. Working group that convened for an editorial and consensus conference in Lyon, France, March 12-16, 2003. Tumours of the Lung. In: *World Health Organization Classification of Tumours. Pathology and Genetics of Tumours of the Lung, Pleura, Thymus and Heart.*

[3] Otto, W.R. (2002) Lung epithelial stem cells. *J Pathol, 197,* 527-535.

[4] Giangreco, A., Groot, K.R., Janes, S.M. (2007) Lung cancer and lung stem cells: strange bedfellows? *Am. J. Respir. Crit. Care Med, 175,* 547-553.

[5] Giangreco, A., Arwert, E.N., Rosewell, I.R., Snyder, J., Watt, F.M., Stripp, B.R. (2009) Stem cells are dispensable for lung homeostasis but restore airways after injury. *Proc. Natl. Acad. Sci. USA, 106,* 9286-9291.

[6] Blanpain, C., Horsley, V., Fuchs, E. Epithelial stem cells: turning over new leaves. (2007) *Cell, 128,* 445-458.

[7] Kitamura, H., Yazawa, T., Shimoyamada, H., Okudela, K., Sato, H. (2008) Molecular and genetic pathogenesis of lung cancer: differences between small-cell and non-small-cell carcinomas. *Open Pathol. J, 2,* 106-114. Doi:10.2174/1874375700802010106

[8] Kitamura, H., Yazawa, T., Sato, H., Okudela, K., Shimoyamada, H. (2009) Small cell lung cancer: significance of RB alterations and TTF-1 expression in its carcinogenesis, phenotype, and biology. *Endcr. Pathol, 20,* 101-107.

References

[9] Nuciforo, P., Fraggetta, F. (2004) Cancer stem cell theory: pathologists' considerations and ruminations about wasting time and wrong evaluations. *J. Clin. Pathol, 7,* 782-783.

[10] Clarke, M.F., Dick, J.E., Dirks, P.B., Eaves, C.J., Jamieson, C.H., Jones, D.L. (2006) Cancer stem cells--perspectives on current status and future directions: AACR Workshop on cancer stem cells. *Cancer Res, 66,* 9339-9344.

[11] Lobo, N.A., Shimono, Y., Qian, D., Clarke, M.F. (2007) The biology of cancer stem cells. *Annu. Rev. Cell Dev. Biol, 23,* 675-699.

[12] Rapp, U.R., Ceteci, F., Schreck, R. (2008) Oncogene-induced plasticity and cancer stem cells. *Cell Cycle, 7,* 45-51.

[13] Kim, C.F., Dirks, P.B. (2008) Cancer and stem cell biology: how tightly intertwined? *Cell Stem Cell, 3,* 147-150.

[14] Yang, Y.M., Chang, J.W. (2008) Current status and issues in cancer stem cell study. *Cancer Invest, 26,* 741-755.

[15] Li, X., Lewis, M.T., Huang, J., Gutierrez, C., Osborne, C.K., Wu, M.F. (2008) Intrinsic resistance of tumorigenic breast cancer cells to chemotherapy. *J. Natl. Cancer Inst, 100,* 672-679.

[16] Li, L., Borodyansky, L., Yang, Y. (2009) Genomic instability en route to and from cancer stem cells. *Cell Cycle, 8,* 1000-1002.

[17] Hill, R.P. (2006) Identifying cancer stem cells in solid tumors: case not proven. *Cancer Res, 66,* 1883-1890.

[18] Kelly, P.N., Dakic, A., Adams, J.M., Nutt, S.L., Strasser, A. (2007) Tumor growth need not be driven by rare cancer stem cells. *Science, 317,* 337.

[19] Lewis, M.T. (2008) Faith, heresy and the cancer stem cell hypothesis. *Future Oncol, 4,* 585-589.

[20] Yoo, M.H., Hatfield, D.L. (2008) The cancer stem cell theory: is it correct? *Mol. Cells, 26,* 514-516.

[21] Vezzoni, L., Parmiani, G. (2008) Limitations of the cancer stem cell theory. *Cytotechnology, 58,* 3-9.

[22] Rowan, K. (2009) Are cancer stem cells real? After four decades, debate still simmers. *J. Natl. Cancer Inst, 101,* 546-547.

[23] Sneddon, J.B., Werb, Z. (2007) Location, location, location: the cancer stem cell niche. *Cell Stem Cell, 1,* 607-611.

[24] Kitamura, H., Okudela, K., Yazawa, T., Sato, H., Shimoyamada, H. (2009) Cancer stem cell: implications in cancer biology and therapy with special reference to lung cancer. *Lung Cancer, 66,* 275-281.

[25] Sung, J.M., Cho, H.J., Yi, H., Lee, C.H., Kim, H.S., Kim, D.K. (2008) Characterization of a stem cell population in lung cancer A549 cells. *Biochem. Biophys. Res. Commun, 371,* 163-167.

[26] Feldmann, G., Dhara, S., Fendrich, V., Bedja, D., Beaty, R., Mullendore, M., Karikari, C., Alvarez, H., Iacobuzio-Donahue, C., Jimeno, A., Gabrielson, K.L., Matsui, W., Maitra, A. (2007) Blockade

of hedgehog signaling pancreatic cancer invasion and metastases: a new paradigm for combination therapy in solid cancers. *Cancer Res, 67,* 2187-96.
[27] Besson, A., Hwang, H.C., Cicero, S., Donovan, S.L., Gurian-West, M., Johnson, D. (2007) Discovery of an oncogenic activity in p27Kip1 that causes stem cell expansion and a multiple tumor phenotype. *Genes Dev, 21,* 1731-1746.
[28] Yin, A.H., Miraglia, S., Zanjani, E.D., Almeida-Porada, G., Ogawa, M., Leary, A.G., et *al.* (1997) AC133, a novel marker for human hematopoietic stem and progenitor cells. *Blood, 90,* 5002-5012.
[29] Wuchter, C., Ratei, R., Spahn, G., Schoch, C., Harbott, J., Schnittger, S., et *al.* (2001) Impact of CD133 (AC133) and CD90 expression analysis for acute leukemia immunophenotyping. *Haematologica, 86,* 154-161.
[30] Shmelkov, S.V., St. Clair, R., Lyden, D., Rafii, S. (2005) AC133/CD133/Prominin-1. *Int. J. Biochem. Cell Biol, 37,* 715-719.
[31] Uchida, N., Buck, D.W., He, D., Reitsma, M.J., Masek, M., Phan, T.V., et *al.* (2000) Direct isolation of human central nervous system stem cells. *Proc. Natl. Acad. Sci. USA, 97,* 14720-14725.
[32] Pötgens, A.J., Bolte, M., Huppertz, B., Kaufmann, P., Frank, H.G. (2001) Human trophoblast contains an intracellular protein reactive with an antibody against CD133--a novel marker for trophoblast. *Placenta, 22,* 39-645.
[33] Salven, P., Mustjoki, S., Alitalo, R., Alitalo, K., Rafii, S. (2003) VEGFR-3 and CD133 identify a population of CD34+ lymphatic/vascular endothelial precursor cells. *Blood, 101,* 168-172.
[34] Richardson, G.D., Robson, C.N., Lang, S.H., Neal, D.E., Maitland, N.J., Collins, A.T. (2004) CD133, a novel marker for human prostatic epithelial stem cells. *Cell Science, 117 pt16,* 3539-3545.
[35] Piechaczek, C. (2001) CD133. *J. Biol. Regul. Homeost Agents, 15,* 101-102.
[36] Yu, Y., Flint, A., Dvorin, E.L., Bischoff, J. (2002) AC133-2, a novel isoform of human AC133 stem cell antigen. *J. Biol. Chem, 277,* 20711-20716.
[37] Marzesco, A.M., Janich, P., Wilsch-Bräuninger, M., Dubreuil, V., Langenfeld, K., Corbeil, D., et *al.* Release of extracellular membrane particles carrying the stem cell marker prominin-1 (CD133) from neural progenitors and other epithelial cells *J. Cell Science, 118 pt13,* 2849-2858.
[38] Taïeb, N., Maresca, M., Guo, X.J., Garmy, N., Fantini, J., Yahi, N. (2009) The first extracellular domain of the tumour stem cell marker CD133 contains an antigenic ganglioside-binding motif. *Cancer Lett, 278,* 164-173.

[39] Choi, D., Lee, H.W., Hur, K.Y., Kim, J.J., Park, G.S., Jang, S.H., et al. Cancer stem cell markers CD133 and CD24 correlate with invasiveness and differentiation in colorectal adenocarcinoma. *World J. Gastroenterol, 15,* 2258-2264.
[40] Ahn, S.M., Goode, R.J., Simpson, R.J. (2008) Stem cell markers: insights from membrane proteomics? *Proteomics, 8,* 4946-4957.
[41] Klonisch, T., Wiechec, E., Hombach-Klonisch, S., Ande, S.R., Wesselborg, S., Schulze-Osthoff, K., *et al.* Cancer stem cell markers in common cancers - therapeutic implications. *Trends Mol. Med, 14,* 450-460.
[42] Eramo, A., Lotti, F., Sette, G., Pilozzi, E., Biffoni, M., Di Virgilio. A., *et al.* (2008), Identification and expansion of the tumorigenic lung cancer stem cell population. *Cell Death Differ, 15,* 504-514.
[43] Wang, J., Sakariassen, P.Ø., Tsinkalovsky, O., Immervoll, H., Bøe, S.O., Svendsen, A., *et al.* (2008) CD133 negative glioma cells form tumors in nude rats and give rise to CD133 positive cells. *Int. J. Cancer, 122,* 761-768.
[44] Ogden, A.T., Waziri, A.E., Lochhead, R.A., Fusco, D., Lopez, K., Ellis, J.A., *et al.* (2008) Identification of A2B5+CD133- tumor-initiating cells in adult human gliomas. *Neurosurgery, 60,* 505-514.
[45] Shmelkov, S.V., Butler, J.M., Hooper, A.T., Hormigo, A., Kushner, J., Milde, T., *et al.* (2008) CD133 expression is not restricted to stem cells, and both CD133+ and CD133- metastatic colon cancer cells initiate tumors. *J. Clin. Invest, 188,* 2111-2120.
[46] Mizrak, D., Brittan, M., Alison, M.R. CD133: molecule of the moment. *J. Pathol, 214,* 3-9.
[47] Bidlingmaier, S., Zhu, X., Liu, B. (2008) The utility and limitations of glycosylated human CD133 epitopes in defining cancer stem cells. *J. Mol. Med, 86,* 1025-1032.
[48] Meng, X., Wang, X., Wang, Y. (2009) More than 45% of A549 and H446 cells are cancer initiating cells: evidence from cloning and tumorigenic analyses. *Oncol. Rep, 12,* 995-1000.
[49] Jiang, F., Qiu, Q., Khanna, A., Todd, N.W., Deepak, J., Xing, L, *et al.* (2009) Aldehyde dehydrogenase 1 is a tumor stem cell-associated marker in lung cancer. *Mol. Cancer Res, 7,* 330-338
[50] Levina, V., Marrangoni, A.M., DeMarco, R., Gorelik, E., Lokshin, A.E. (2008) Drug-selected human lung cancer stem cells: cytokine network, tumorigenic and metastatic properties. *PLoS ONE, 2,* e3077.
[51] Chen, Y.C., Hsu, H.S., Chen, Y.W., Tsai, T.H., How, C.K., Wang, C.Y., *et al.* (2008) Oct-4 expression maintained cancer stem-like properties in lung cancer-derived CD133-positive cells. *PLoS ONE, 3,* e2637.
[52] Jiang, T., Collins, B.J., Jin, N., Watkins, D.N., Brock, M.V., Matsui, W., *et al.* (2009) Achaete-scute complex homologue 1 regulates

tumor-initiating capacity in human small cell lung cancer. *Cancer Res, 69,* 845-854.

[53] Ito, T., Udaka, N., Okudela, K., Yazawa, T., Kitamura, H. (2003) Mechanisms of neuroendocrine differentiation in pulmonary neuroendocrine cells and small cell carcinoma. *Endocr. Pathol, 14,* 133-139.

[54] Goodell, M.A., Brose, K., Paradis, G., Conner, A.S., Mulligan, R.C. (1996) Isolation and functional properties of murine hematopoietic stem cells that are replicating in vivo. *J. Exp. Med, 183,* 1797-1806.

[55] Wu, C., Alman, B.A. Side population cells in human cancers. *Cancer Lett, 268,* 1-9.

[56] Hirschmann-Jax, C., Foster, A.E., Wulf, G.G., Nuchtern, J.G., Jax, T.W., Gobel, U., *et al.* (2004) A distinct "side population" of cells with high drug efflux capacity in human tumor cells. *Proc. Natl. Acad. Sci. USA, 101,* 14228-14233.

[57] Hirschmann-Jax, C., Foster, A.E., Wulf, G.G., Goodell, M.A., Brenner, M.K. (2005) A distinct "side population" of cells in human tumor cells: implications for tumor biology and therapy. *Cell Cycle,* 4, 203-205

[58] Zhou, S., Schuetz, J.D., Bunting, K.D., Colapietro, A.M., Sampath, J., Morris, J.J., *et al.* (2001) The ATP binding cassette transporter Bcrp1/ABCG2 is expressed in a wide variety of stem cells and is a molecular determinant of the side-population phenotype. *Nat. Med, 7,* 1028-1034.

[59] Telford, W.G., Bradford, J., Godfrey, W., Robey, R.W., Bates, S.E. (2007) Side population analysis using a violet-excited cell-permeable DNA dye. *Stem Cells, 25,* 1029-1036.

[60] Ho MM, Ng AV, Lam S, Hung JY. Side population in human lung cancer cell lines and tumors is enriched with stem-like cancer cells. *Cancer Res.* 2007; 67:4827-4833.

[61] Sophos, N.A., Vasiliou, V. (2003) Aldehyde dehydrogenase gene superfamily: the 2009 update. *Chem. Biol. Interact, 143-144, 5-22.*

[62] Huang, E.H., Hynes, M.J., Zhang, T., Ginestier, C., Dontu, G., Appelman, H., *et al.* (2009) Aldehyde dehydrogenase 1 is a marker for normal and malignant human colonic stem cells (SC) and tracks SC overpopulation during colon tumorigenesis. *Cancer Res, 69,* 3382-3389.

[63] Jones, R.J., Barber, J.P., Vala, M.S., Collector, M.I., Kaufmann, S.H., Ludeman, S.M., *et al.* (1995) Assessment of aldehyde dehydrogenase in viable cells. *Blood, 85,* 2742-2746.

[64] Armstrong, L., Stojkovic, M., Dimmick, I., Ahmad, S., Stojkovic, P., Hole, N., *et al.* (2004) Phenotypic characterization of murine primitive hematopoietic progenitor cells isolated on basis of aldehyde dehydroganse activity. *Stem Cells, 22,* 1142-1151.

[65] Corti, S., Locatelli, F., Papadimitriou, D., Donadoni, C., Salani, S., Del Bo, R., et al. (2006) Identification of a primitive brain-derived neural stem cell population based on aldehyde dehydrogenase activity. *Stem Cells, 24*, 975-985.
[66] Ginestier, C., Hur, M.H., Charafe-Jauffret, E., Monville, F., Dutcher, J., Brown, M., et al. (2007) ALDH1 is a marker of normal and malignant human mammary stem cells and a predictor of poor clinical outcome. *Cell Stem Cell, 1*, 555-567.
[67] Dylla, S.J., Beviglia, L., Park, I.K., Chartier, C., Raval, J., Ngan, L., et al. (2008) Colorectal cancer stem cells are enriched in xenogeneic tumors following chemotherapy. *PLoS ONE, 3*, e2428.
[68] Storms, R.W., Trujillo, A.P., Springer, J.B., Shah, L., Colvin, O.M., Ludeman, S.M., et al. (1999) Isolation of primitive human hematopoietic progenitors on the basis of aldehyde dehydrogenase activity. *Proc. Natl. Acad. Sci. USA, 96*, 9118-9123.
[69] Koch, L.K., Zhou, H., Ellinger, J., Biermann, K., Höller, T., von Rücker, A., et al. (2008) Stem cell marker expression in small cell lung carcinoma and developing lung tissue. *Hum. Pathol, 39*, 1597-1605.
[70] Lanza, F., Healy, L., Sutherland, D.R. Structural and functional features of the CD34 antigen: an update. *J. Biol. Regul. Homeost Agents, 15*, 1-13.
[71] Nielsen, J.S., McNagny, K.M. (2008) Novel functions of the CD34 family. *J. Cell Sci, 121pt22*, 3683-92.
[72] Doyonnas, R., Nielsen, J.S., Chelliah, S., Drew, E., Hara, T., Miyajima, A., McNagny, K.M. (2005) *Blood, 105*, 4170-4178.
[73] Gutova, M., Najbauer, J., Gevorgyan, A., Metz, M.Z., Weng, Y., Shih, C.C., et al. (2007) Identification of uPAR-positive chemoresistant cells in small cell lung cancer. *PLoS ONE, 2*, e243.
[74] Alfano, D., Franco, P., Vocca, I., Gambi, N., Pisa, V., Mancini, A., Caputi, M., Carriero, M.V., Iaccarino, I., Stoppelli, M.P. (2009) The urokinase plasminogen activator and its receptor: role in cell growth and apoptosis. *Thromb Haemost, 93*, 205-211.
[75] Van der Flier, L.G., Clevers, H. (2009) Stem cells, self-renewal, and differentiation in the intestinal epithelium. *Annu. Rev. Physiol, 71*, 5.1-5.20.
[76] Liao, X., Siu, M.K., Au, C.W., Chan, Q.K., Chan, H.Y., Wong, E.S., et al. (2009) Aberrant activation of hedgehog signaling pathway contributes to endometrial carcinogenesis through β-catenin. *Mod. Pathol, 22*, 839-847.
[77] Watkins, D.N., Berman, D.M., Burkholder, S.G., Wang, B., Beachy, P.A., Baylin, S.B. (2003) Hedgehog signalling within airway epithelial progenitors and in small-cell lung cancer. *Nature, 422*, 313-317.

[78] Yagui-Beltrán, A., He, B., Jablons, D.M. (2008) The role of cancer stem cells in neoplasia of the lung: past, present and future. *Clin. Transl Oncol, 10,* 719-725.
[79] Peacock, C.D., Watkins, D.N. (2008) Cancer stem cells and the ontogeny of lung cancer. *J. Clin. Oncol, 26,* 2883-2889.
[80] Lemjabbar-Alaoui, H., Dasari, V., Sidhu, S.S., Mengistab, A., Finkbeiner, W., Gallup, M., et al. (2006) Wnt and Hedgehog are critical mediators of cigarette smoke-induced lung cancer. *PLoS ONE, 1,* e93.
[81] Alison, M.R., Islam, S. (2009) Attributes of adult stem cells. *J. Pathol, 217,* 144-160.
[82] Polakis, P. (2000) Wnt signaling and cancer. *Genes Dev, 14,* 1837-1851.
[83] Reya, T., Clevers, H. (2005) Wnt signalling in stem cells and cancer. *Nature, 434,* 843-850.
[84] Valk-Lingbeek, M.E., Bruggenman, S.W.M., van Lohuizen, M. (2004) Stem cell and cancer: poly-comb connection. *Cell, 118,* 409-418.
[85] Dovey, J.S., Zacharek, S.J., Kim, C.F., Lees, J.A. (2008) Bmi1 is critical for lung tumorigenesis and bronchioalveolar stem cell expansion. *Proc. Natl. Acad. Sci. USA. 105,* 11857-11862.
[86] Ovitt, C.E., Schöler, H.R. (1998) The molecular biology of Oct-4 in the early mouse embryo. *Mol. Hum. Reprod, 4,* 1021-1031.
[87] Basak, S.K., Veena, M.S., Oh, S., Huang, G., Srivatsan, E., Huang, M., Sharma, S., Batra, R.K. (2009) The malignant pleural effusion as a model to investigate intratumoral heterogeneity in lung cancer. *PLoS One, 4,* e5884.
[88] Collins, A.T., Berry, P.A., Hyde, C., Stower, M.J., Maitland, N.J. (2005) Prospective identification of tumorigenic prostate cancer stem cells. *Cancer Res, 65,* 10946-10951.
[89] Annabi, B., Lachambre, M.P., Plouffe, K., Sartelet, H., Béliveau, R. (2009) Modulation of invasive properties of CD133(+) glioblastoma stem cells: a role for MT1-MMP in bioactive lysophospholipid signaling. *Mol. Carcinog, 48,* 910-919.
[90] Li, L., Neaves, W.B. (2006) Normal stem cells and cancer stem cells: the niche matters. *Cancer Res, 66,* 4553-4557.
[91] Hilbe, W., Dirnhofer, S., Oberwasserlechner, F., Schmid, T., Gunsilius, E., Hilbe, G., et al. (2004) CD133 positive endothelial progenitor cells contribute to the tumour vasculature in non-small cell lung cancer. *J. Clin. Pathol, 57,* 965-969.
[92] Moreb, J.S., Baker, H.V., Chang, L.J., Amaya, M., Lopez, M.C., Ostmark, B., Chou, W. (2008) ALDH isozymes downregulation affects cell growth, cell motility and gene expression in lung cancer cells. *Mol. Cancer, 7,* 87.

[93] Moreb, J.S., Zucali, J.R., Ostmark, B., Benson, N.A. (2007) Heterogeneity of aldehyde dehydrogenase expression in lung cancer cell lines is revealed by Aldefluor flow cytometry-based assay. *Cytometry B Clin. Cytom, 72*, 281-9.
[94] Moreb, J.S. (2008) Aldehyde dehydrogenase as a marker for stem cells. *Curr. Stem Cell Res. Ther, 3*, 237-46.
[95] Ucar, D., Cogle, C.R., Zucali, J.R., Ostmark, B., Scott, E.W., Zori, R., *et al.* (2009) Aldehyde dehydrogenase activity as a functional marker for lung cancer. *Chem. Biol. Interact, 178*, 48-55.
[96] Patel, M., Lu, L., Zander, D.S., Sreerama, L., Coco, D., Moreb, J.S. (2008) ALDH1A1 and ALDH3A1 expression in lung cancers: correlation with histologic type and potential precursors. *Lung Cancer, 59*, 340-349.
[97] Carpentino, J.E., Hynes, M.J., Appelman, H.D., Zheng, T., Steindler, D.A., Scott, E.W., Huang, E.H. (2008) Aldehyde dehydrogenase-expressing colon stem cells contribute to tumorigenesis in the transition from colitis to cancer. *Cancer Res, 69*, 8208-8215.
[98] Christ, O., Lucke, K., Imren, S., Leung, K., Hamilton, M., Eaves, A., Smith, C., Eaves, C. (2007) Improved purification of hematopoietic stem cells based on their elevated aldehyde dehydrogenase activity. *Haematologica, 92*, 1165-1172.
[99] Sisson, J.H. (2007) Alcohol and airways function in health and disease. *Alcohol, 41*, 293-307.
[100] Moriwaki, Y., Yamamoto, T., Higashino, K. (1997) Distribution and pathophysiologic role of molybdenum-containing enzymes. *Histol Histopathol, 12*, 513-524.
[101] Yin SJ. Alcohol dehydrogenase: enzymology and metabolism. *Alcohol Alcohol Suppl.* 1994;2:113-9.
[102] Cozens, A.L., Yezzi, M.J., Kunzelmann, K., Ohrui, T., Chin, L., Eng, K., Finkbeiner, W.E., Widdicombe, J.H., Gruenert, D.C. CFTR expression and chloride secretion in polarized immortal human bronchial epithelial cells. *Am. J. Respir. Cell Mol. Biol, 10*, 38-47.
[103] Masuda, A., Kondo, M., Saito, T., Yatabe, Y., Kobayashi, T., Okamoto, M., Suyama, M., Takahashi, T., Takahashi, T. (1997) Establishment of human peripheral lung epithelial cell lines (HPL1) retaining differentiated characteristics and responsiveness to epidermal growth factor, hepatocyte growth factor, and transforming growth factor β1. *Cancer Res, 57*, 4898-4904.
[104] Okudela, K., Hayashi, H., Ito, T., Yazawa, T., Suzuki, T., Nakane, Y., Sato, H., Ishi, H., KeQin, X., Masuda, A., Takahashi, T., Kitamura, H. (2004) K-ras gene mutation enhances motility of immortalized airway cells and lung adenocarcinoma cells via Akt activation: possible contribution to non-invasive expansion of lung adenocarcinoma. *Am. J. Pathol, 164*, 91-100.

[105] Deshusses JM, Burgess JA, Scherl A, Wenger Y, Walter N, Converset V, Paesano S, Corthals GL, Hochstrasser DF, Sanchez JC. (2003) Exploitation of specific properties of trifluoroethanol for extraction and separation of membrane proteins. *Proteomics, 3,* 1418-1424.

[106] Zhan X, Desiderio DM. (2003) Spot volume vs. amount of protein loaded onto a gel: a detailed, statistical comparison of two gel electrophoresis systems. *Electrophoresis, 24,* 1818-1833.

Index

A

acetylation, 41
acid, 17, 28
acute leukemia, 51
ADC, ix, 1, 3, 33, 34, 36, 40, 42, 45, 46
adenocarcinoma, ix, 1, 33, 34, 36, 42, 45, 46, 56
adult stem cells, 55
aggressiveness, 1, 3, 14
airway epithelial cells, 33, 43
airways, 49, 56
aldehydes, 17
alveoli, 1
alveolus, 45
amino, 13, 39
amino acid, 13, 39
amino acids, 39
anchorage, 25
antibody, 19, 32, 34, 42, 43, 45, 46, 51
anti-cancer, 14, 23
antigen, 13, 17, 45, 51, 54
APC, 22
apoptosis, 19, 54
ATP, ix, 3, 11, 15, 53

B

base, 39
base pair, 39
biological behavior, 2, 3, 47
bone, ix, 15, 23
bone marrow, 15
brain, 13, 53
brain tumor, 13
breast cancer, 13, 50
bronchial epithelial cells, 21, 22, 33, 56
bronchus, 45

C

cancer, ix, 1, 2, 3, 11, 13, 14, 21, 23, 25, 26, 27, 28, 33, 43, 45, 47, 48, 49, 50, 52, 53, 54, 55, 56
cancer cells, 1, 14, 21, 28, 33, 43, 47, 48, 53
carcinogenesis, 2, 21, 49, 54
carcinoma, vii, ix, 1, 11, 33, 34, 36, 42, 45, 46, 52, 54
cDNA, ix, 33, 39
cell biology, 2, 48, 50
cell line, 3, 8, 9, 10, 11, 14, 16, 23, 27, 28, 29, 31, 32, 33, 34, 35, 36, 39, 41, 42, 43, 47, 48, 53, 55, 56
cell lines, 3, 8, 9, 10, 14, 16, 24, 27, 28, 29, 31, 32, 33, 34, 35, 36, 39, 43, 47, 48, 53, 55, 56
cell surface, 19
central nervous system, 13, 51

chemiluminescence, 34, 42
chemotherapeutic agent, 15
chemotherapy, 3, 28, 50, 54
cigarette smoke, 21, 22, 43, 55
City, 33, 48
classification, 1
clonality, 24
clone, 32, 33, 34, 42, 45
cloning, 14, 16, 39, 52
coding, 40
colitis, 56
colon, 52, 53, 56
colon cancer, 52
colorectal adenocarcinoma, 51
colorectal cancer, 13
combination therapy, 50
communication, 25
conference, 49
consensus, 13, 40, 49
consent, 45
contamination, 15
correlation, 28, 56
correlations, 27
CSCs, v, 2, 3, 7, 13, 14, 15, 21, 22, 23, 24, 25, 26, 27, 28, 47, 48
culture, 21, 24
culture conditions, 24
cures, 3
cytometry, 55

D

deaths, 1
degradation, 22
deoxyribonucleic acid, ix
detectable, 31
detection, 45, 46
detection system, 45, 46
disorder, 39
diversity, 1
DNA, 15, 53
drug efflux, 53
drugs, 14, 23

E

electrophoresis, 34, 42, 57
emission, 37
encoding, 39
endothelial cells, 26
enzymatic activity, 27, 29, 48
enzyme, 17
enzymes, 17, 28, 56
epidemiology, 49
epidermis, 21
epithelia, 1, 21, 44, 45, 48
epithelial cells, 13, 21, 25, 43, 51
epithelium, 54
etiology, 7, 49
evidence, 5, 25, 28, 41, 52
excitation, 37
extraction, 34, 56
extracts, 34

F

fluorescence, ix, 15, 36, 47
force, 2
formation, 24
France, 49

G

gel, 34, 42, 57
gene expression, 55
genes, 1, 2, 15, 17, 24
genetic alteration, 2
genomic instability, 2
Germany, 40
gland, 1, 21
glioblastoma, 55
glioma, 52
glycosylation, 41
graph, 34, 45
growth, ix, 2, 50, 54, 55, 56
growth factor, ix, 2, 56

H

health, 56
hematopoietic stem cells, 15, 17, 19, 53, 56
heterogeneity, 1, 2, 7, 48, 55
homeostasis, 5, 49
human, 3, 13, 15, 17, 21, 22, 23, 32, 34, 51, 52, 53, 54, 56
human genome, 17
hydrogen, 45
hydrogen peroxide, 45
hypothesis, 47, 50

I

identification, 1, 24, 55
immunocompromised, 13
immunohistochemistry, 26, 43, 45
in vitro, 3, 14, 23, 24, 27, 43, 47
in vivo, 14, 24, 27, 43, 47, 48, 53
inhibitor, 3, 36
initiation, 7, 26
integration, ix, 11, 23
integrin, 13, 25
intervention, 1
intestine, 1
Islam, 55
isolation, 16, 17, 24, 51
isozymes, 27, 28, 43, 55
issues, 28, 50

J

Japan, 33, 42, 45, 48

K

kill, 3

L

lead, 2, 3, 11, 15
legend, 34, 37, 40
lesions, 2
lung cancer, 1, 2, 3, 7, 9, 13, 14, 16, 23, 24, 26, 27, 28, 31, 32, 34, 36, 39, 43, 45, 47, 48, 49, 50, 52, 53, 54, 55, 56

M

machinery, 47
majority, 1, 19, 23
malignant tumors, 13
materials, 33, 34, 37, 42, 45
matter, iv, 7, 25
measurement, 17
membranes, 34, 42
mesenchyme, 21
messenger ribonucleic acid, ix
metabolic pathways, 28
metabolism, 28, 56
metastasis, 3
mice, 13, 15, 21, 22, 23
migration, 19
Ministry of Education, 48
MMP, 55
models, 25
modifications, 41
molecular biology, 55
molecular targeting, 48
molecular weight, 42
molecules, 3
molybdenum, 56
motif, 51
mRNA, v, ix, 29, 31, 32, 33, 35, 39, 40, 47, 48
mucosa, 21
multipotent, 28
mutation, 22, 39, 41, 56
mutations, 19

N

National Institute of Mental Health, 34
neuroendocrine cells, 52
nuclei, 45
nucleotide sequence, 39

nucleus, 22

O

oncogenes, 2, 19
ovarian cancer, 13
overpopulation, 53
oxidation, 17

P

Pacific, 33
pancreatic cancer, 3, 13, 50
parallel, 44, 48
pathogenesis, 3, 7, 47, 49
pathology, 7
pathways, 2, 3, 19, 21, 23
PCR, ix, 9, 29, 31, 33, 40
penicillin, 33
phenotype, 3, 15, 16, 27, 49, 51, 53
phosphorylation, 41
photographs, 45
physicians, 2
plasmid, 40
plasminogen, ix, 11, 19, 54
plasticity, 2, 50
pleura, 49
pleural effusion, 55
polyacrylamide, 34, 42
polymerase, ix, 29
polymerase chain reaction, ix, 29
polymorphism, 39
population, ix, 3, 11, 14, 15, 19, 23, 47, 50, 51, 52, 53
post-transcriptional regulation, 39
precursor cells, 13, 51
preparation, iv
prevention, 19
primary tumor, 47
progenitor cells, 2, 3, 5, 7, 13, 26, 51, 53, 55
prognosis, 1, 3
proliferation, 2, 17
promoter, 40
prostate cancer, 13, 55

protein structure, 41
proteins, 23, 29, 32, 42, 43, 56
proteolysis, 19
proteomics, 51
purification, 56
purity, 16

R

radio, 14, 23
reactions, 33
reading, 39
reagents, 33
real time, 28
receptors, 21
recommendations, iv
recurrence, 3, 15
repair, 5
researchers, 2
resistance, 3, 15, 16, 50
response, 5, 43
responsiveness, 1, 56
retinoblastoma, ix
retinol, 17, 28
RNA, ix, 33
rodents, 13

S

scatter, 36
secretion, 56
serum, 33, 45
services, iv
signal transduction, 2
signaling pathway, 2, 3, 21, 22, 23, 27, 54
signalling, 54, 55
signals, 21, 25, 26
siRNA, ix, 28
skin, 1
sodium, 34, 42
solid tumors, 50
spectrophotometry, 28
squamous cell, ix, 1, 33, 34, 36, 45, 46

squamous cell carcinoma, ix, 1, 33, 34, 36, 45, 46
standard deviation, 45
state, 3
stem cells, 1, 2, 7, 13, 15, 17, 21, 23, 24, 25, 26, 28, 48, 49, 50, 51, 52, 53, 54, 55, 56
stress, 43
structure, 40
substitution, 39
substrate, 17
sulfate, 34, 42
surgical resection, 45

T

target, 1, 2, 3, 48
technology, 36
therapy, 2, 15, 48, 50, 53
thymus, 49
thyroid, ix, 2
tissue, 1, 2, 8, 9, 11, 21, 24, 27, 45, 54
tobacco, 2, 5
tobacco smoke, 2, 5
toxic substances, 5
toxicity, 15
TP53, ix, 2
tracks, 53
transcription, ix, 2, 22, 24, 29
transcription factors, 22
transduction, 32, 46
transformation, 2, 22
transforming growth factor, 56
treatment, 3, 14, 23, 45, 48
tumor, ix, 2, 15, 16, 23, 26, 45, 46, 51, 52, 53
tumor cells, 53
tumor growth, 26
tumorigenesis, 53, 55, 56
tumors, 13, 43, 45, 48, 52, 53, 54

U

urokinase, ix, 11, 19, 54
USA, 49, 51, 53, 54, 55

V

variables, 15
vasculature, 26, 55
vector, 40

W

Western blot, 9, 17, 27, 28, 29, 32, 34, 35, 41, 42, 43
Wnt signaling, 21, 22, 55
World Health Organization, 49
worldwide, 1

X

X-axis, 36
xenotransplantation, 13

Y

Y-axis, 36